DRUG ABUSE:
A CRIMINAL JUSTICE PRIMER

GLENCOE PRESS CRIMINAL JUSTICE SERIES

Allen/Simonsen: **Corrections in America: An Introduction**

Bloomquist: **Marijuana: The Second Trip**

Brandstatter/Hyman: **Fundamentals of Law Enforcement**

Brandstatter/Radelet: **Police and Community Relations**

Eldefonso: **Issues in Corrections**

Eldefonso: **Readings in Criminal Justice**

Eldefonso/Coffey: **Process and Impact of Justice**

Eldefonso/Coffey: **Process and Impact of Juvenile Justice System**

Eldefonso/Hartinger: **Control, Treatment, and Rehabilitation of Juvenile Offenders**

Engel/DeGreen/Rebo: **The Justice Game: A Simulation**

Gourley: **Effective Municipal Police Organization**

Koga/Nelson: **The Koga Method: Police Weaponless Control and Defense Techniques**

Koga/Nelson: **The Koga Method: Police Baton Techniques**

LeGrande: **The Basic Processes of Criminal Justice**

Lentini: **Vice and Narcotics Control**

McArthur: **Police Patrol Pointers**

Melnicoe/Mennig: **Elements of Police Supervision**

Nelson: **Preliminary Investigation and Police Reporting: A Complete Guide to Police Written Communication**

Radelet: **The Police and the Community**

Radelet: **The Police and the Community: Studies**

Roberts/Bristow: **An Introduction to Modern Police Firearms**

Waddington: **Arrest, Search, and Seizure**

Wicks/Platt: **Drug Abuse: A Criminal Justice Primer**

Williams: **Narcotics and Drug Dependence**

General Editor:

G. DOUGLAS GOURLEY

Inspector (Ret.), LA Police Department
Chairman, Department of Criminal Justice
California State University at Los Angeles
Los Angeles, California

DRUG ABUSE: A CRIMINAL JUSTICE PRIMER

Robert J. Wicks
Clinical Senior Instructor
College of Allied Health Professions
Hahnemann Medical College and Hospital

Jerome J. Platt
Associate Professor and Associate Director of
Research and Evaluation
Department of Mental Health Sciences
Hahnemann Medical College and Hospital

GLENCOE PRESS
A division of Benziger Bruce & Glencoe, Inc.
Beverly Hills

Collier Macmillan Publishers
London

This book is dedicated to our parents

Printed in the United States of America

GLENCOE PRESS
A division of Benziger Bruce & Glencoe, Inc.
8701 Wilshire Boulevard
Beverly Hills, California 90211
Collier Macmillan Canada, Ltd.

Library of Congress Card Number: 76-4027

1 2 3 4 5 6 7 8 9 KPt 80 79 78 77 76

Contents

Preface

CRIMINAL JUSTICE PERSONNEL are painfully aware of the scope of the illegal drug problem. Not only are these men and women aware of the effects of drug abuse in terms of wasted lives and human suffering, but it is their responsibility to investigate drug abuse cases and to attempt to eradicate or control the numerous criminal activities that are related to drug processing, trafficking, and sales.

Consequently, it is imperative that police officers, sheriffs, correction officers, military police, state and federal investigators, and criminal justice college majors have a basic knowledge of the various drugs of abuse. In addition, these professionals must have an understanding of the general approach, as well as the specific law enforcement techniques, employed by the criminal justice system to combat drug abuse.

To obtain this vital information on drugs and the problems related to their abuse, professionals and students have taken courses and read books on the general subject of drug abuse. Too many times, however, they have been frustrated in their search for a single book that examines basic information on drugs, the nature of drug abuse, and the relationship of drug abuse with the criminal justice system. For the most part, drug abuse books currently available are either too cumbersome, too technical, or too laden with explanations of law enforcement procedures.

Drug Abuse: A Criminal Justice Primer has been specifically written to fulfill the need for a concise but thorough single-volume discussion of drugs use and abuse. The authors recognize that if criminal justice professionals are to deal effectively with the problems of illegal drug use, they must have a basic, nontechnical understanding of the various drugs of abuse.

The book has two main divisions—one on the drugs themselves, the other on treatment, prevention, and criminal investigation. Part 1, ''Drug Use and Commonly Abused Drugs,'' examines in detail the major drugs of abuse—alcohol, heroin, tranquilizers, marijuana, hallucinogens, amphetamines, and cocaine. Each of the drugs is discussed in terms of patterns of use, effects and side effects, and addiction, when applicable.

Part 2, ''Treatment, Enforcement and Prevention, and Investigation'' takes a close look at important aspects of treatment for the drug abuser and prevention and investigation methods employed by law enforcement personnel. The chapters on prevention and investigation will be of special value to criminal justice personnel, for in these chapters the reader will find specific information on legal measures to control drug abuse and drug traffic and the procedures and techniques of investigating illegal drug use.

In preparing a concise introductory volume on any subject, choices must be made as to what should or should not be included. Although this book is no exception, the authors are convinced that it will prove useful as a comprehensive first text on drug abuse for criminal justice personnel. It should be kept in mind that this book is intended to serve as a point of departure, not an end, in your understanding of drug abuse and its relationship to law enforcement. Viewed in this light, officers and other criminal justice personnel will find this book extremely useful as a course text or as an addition to their professional library.

Robert J. Wicks
Jerome J. Platt

Acknowledgments

OFTEN, IN THE PREPARATION of a book, many people contribute either directly or indirectly to its development. This has been particularly the case in the writing of this book, and we wish to express our sincere appreciation to these people.

First, we wish to thank our wives, Michaele Wicks and Kay Platt, for their patience and help. We also wish to acknowledge the information, comments, research assistance, and general support which were provided in many varied ways by Special Agent James Kibble, Capt. Arthur Cinotti, Rev. James R. Harvey, Janis Clarke, Barbara Williams, Judith Baker, and Sonja Fox. Grace Verna, who did an outstanding job of typing and otherwise preparing the final form of the manuscript, deserves our special thanks.

In acknowledging contributions, we would also like to thank Hahnemann Medical College and Hospital's Mental Health Sciences Department, which operates under the direction of Dr. Israel Zwerling; the general impetus given this work by the department cannot be overstated.

Finally, the authors wish to express their gratitude to Dr. John J. Bellizzi, Executive Director of the International Narcotic Enforcement Officers Association, for providing essential information on his organization, and to the Christopher D. Smithers Foundation and Alcoholics Anonymous World Services, Inc. for granting us permission to quote from their publications.

Part 1

DRUG USE AND COMMONLY ABUSED DRUGS

Chapter 1
Drug Use and Drug Abuse

From the earliest days of civilization, certain substances have been widely known for their ability to influence the way a person thinks, feels, behaves, and perceives the world. Such substances have been used by people all over the world for thousands of years. Alcoholic beverages, for example, are known to have been in use as many as 8,500 years ago, and some authorities suggest that their use may date back even further than that.[1] There is also reason to believe that certain hallucinogenic substances* may have been in use almost as long ago as alcohol was—particularly in religious ceremonies.

Thus, the use of drugs to attain altered states of consciousness is not a new phenomenon. Neither, apparently, is drug *abuse,* for, as will be discussed in Chapter 2, long ago it became necessary for societies to pass laws regulating the use of alcohol.

If drug abuse is an age-old problem, it is also a very contemporary one, visible at all levels of society. Its victims range from the alcoholic on skid row to the young narcotics addict who is admitted to a hospital emergency room to be treated for an overdose of heroin to the housewife who uses amphetamines to "pep" her up. As one indication of the extent of the drug abuse problem in the United States, it was estimated in 1973 that there were as many as 819,000 *narcotics* addicts alone.[2] By now this figure may have risen to over 1,000,000. Of particular relevance (and concern) to criminal justice personnel are the findings of one of the authors of this book who, during the past eight years, has kept a close watch on drug abuse patterns among new admissions to the New Jersey Reformatory Complex—an institution through which approximately 80 percent of the state's male offenders aged 15 to 30 pass when remanded to a correctional facility.[3] In 1968, documented use of dangerous drugs was present in some 37 percent of new admissions, with some two-thirds of this number being heroin users. In July, 1971, an all-time high was reached when documented histories of drug use were found to be present in 80 percent of new admissions, the overwhelming majority of whom (73 percent) were using heroin.

*Hallucinogenic substances have the ability to strongly influence the way we perceive the world as well as the way we feel. Currently used hallucinogens include lysergic acid diethylamide (LSD-25), mescaline, and marijuana.

Despite the fact that by 1975 these figures had declined somewhat (to 76 percent, of which 48.5 percent were using heroin), they nevertheless make a strong case for the need for experienced personnel within the criminal justice system, individuals who are knowledgeable about the various drugs of abuse—including the manner in which they are abused and their characteristic effects. This chapter will examine the nature of drug abuse and present some general background on how drugs produce their effects. Many of the concepts and issues touched upon here will be treated at greater length in subsequent chapters.

What Is Drug Abuse?

Dr. Jerome H. Jaffe, former Director of the White House Special Action Office for Drug Abuse, defines drug abuse as "the use, usually by self-administration, of any drug in a manner that deviates from the approved medical or social patterns within a given culture."[4] Thus, according to this definition, practically any drug has a potential for abuse. However, for the purposes of our discussion, we will focus only on those drugs that produce appreciable changes in mood and behavior. Included in this group are all the substances listed in Table 1.1, as well as others that are not listed but that nonetheless have a potential for abuse.

It should be pointed out that not all abused drugs are necessarily illegal. Alcohol, for example, is not an illegal drug, although its use is regulated. Likewise, solvents such as cleaning fluids or glues may be purchased legally, and such drugs as barbiturates, amphetamines, and tranquilizers are not illegal when obtained through a physician's prescription.

Commonly Abused Drugs

The major drugs of abuse can be classified into four different categories: *depressants, stimulants, narcotics,* and *hallucinogens*. The depressants are drugs that act by depressing the central nervous system. Among the most common depressant drugs are alcohol, the sedatives, and tranquilizers. The stimulants, in contrast, are drugs that act by stimulating the central nervous system. The most commonly abused stimulants are the amphetamines and cocaine. Among narcotics, the opiates, which are derived from the opium poppy, relieve pain, deaden feelings, cause drowsiness, and generally sap the user's energy. Among the most common opiates are opium, heroin, and morphine. There also exist manufactured or synthetic narcotics which produce essentially the same effects as the naturally occurring opiates. An example of such a synthetic narcotic is methadone. Finally, the hallucinogens, so named because of their ability to produce hallucinations, include many substances, the most common of which are marijuana and LSD. All of these drugs and others will be discussed in greater detail in subsequent chapters. (See Table 1.1.)

Reasons for Drug Abuse

Drug abuse may develop for any number of reasons. But, generally speaking, the most common causes of drug abuse fall into two major categories. The first category includes the reasons for *initial* drug use, whereas the second category includes the reasons for *continued* drug use. Although many of the reasons belonging to the first category overlap into the second category—for example, the influence of friends—others, such as the need to continue drug use in order to prevent the occurrence of withdrawal symptoms, belong exclusively to the second.

Initial drug use may occur for one or more of the following reasons:

1. To escape from an unpleasant reality by "dulling" one's senses.
2. To obtain a state of heightened pleasure or euphoria.
3. To induce relaxation, or to reduce a high level of tension or anxiety.
4. To gain membership in the "in-group."
5. To relieve physical pain.
6. To bolster a poor self-image, perhaps by becoming a member of a drug culture.
7. To enhance creativity.
8. To have a new and novel experience.

As can be clearly seen, at least two of the reasons listed above might constitute legitimate grounds for a physician to prescribe a drug which, in the hands of the wrong patient, could later lead to abuse. For example, it would not be inappropriate for a physician to prescribe tranquilizers for a patient suffering from a constant state of anxiety, or to administer a narcotic to one experiencing unusual pain. But problems arise because some individuals seem to develop a desire for the secondary effects of the drug (such as the euphoria afforded by narcotics), even after the initial need for the drug has been alleviated. The patient who continues to use tranquilizers, even though the need is no longer evident, is a common example of such an individual.

Some persons seek out drugs specifically for the mood-changing qualities they possess. For instance, some drugs are reputed to enhance sexual ability, or to produce a "fantastic high"; others are believed to enhance creativity or to increase self-awareness.

Other factors that may contribute to initial drug use include the influence of friends or the use of a drug as a means of gaining acceptance into a particular group. Contrary to popular belief, however, most young people begin using drugs—particularly "hard" drugs such as heroin—not because they are encouraged to do so by older youths, but because they hope that by using the drug they will be able to share in the older group's activities.[5] Similarly, individuals who use hallucinogens often do so not because of coercion but because they themselves see the use of the drug as a badge identifying them as members of a

TABLE 1.1 SUMMARY TABLE OF ABUSED DRUGS

DRUG	CHAPTER	LEGITIMATE MEDICAL USES	METHODS OF USE	TYPICAL DOSE	DURATION OF ACTION
Alcohol (depressant)	2	External antiseptic, sedative	Swallowed in beverage form	Varies, depending on type of beverage	Depends on amount consumed
Heroin (narcotic)	4	None	Usually injected under skin or into vein or muscle; sometimes swallowed or sniffed	"Bag" containing 5–10% pure heroin	4 hours
Opium (narcotic)	4	None	Usually smoked in pipe; may be eaten	Several pipefuls	4 hours
Morphine (narcotic)	4	Pain reliever	Swallowed or, more often, injected under the skin or into the muscle or vein	15 mg	6 hours
Codeine (narcotic)	4	Pain reliever, cough depressant, relief of diarrhea	Swallowed or injected	30 mg	4 hours
Methadone (synthetic narcotic)	4	Relief of pain, narcotic antagonist	Swallowed in tablet or liquid form, or injected	5–15 mg	4–6 hours
Cannabis: Marijuana and hashish (euphoriants/hallucinogens)	5	None	Smoked in cigarettes or pipe; sometimes eaten or sniffed	1–2 cigarettes or pipefuls	4 hours

SOURCES: "Drug Abuse Products Reference Chart," Smith, Kline, & French Laboratories; *Drugs of Abuse,* Bureau of Narcotics and Dangerous Drugs, U.S. Department of Justice; *Resource Book for Drug Abuse Education,* National Institute of Mental Health.

TOLERANCE	POTENTIAL FOR DEVELOPMENT OF PHYSICAL DEPENDENCE	PSYCHOLOGICAL DEPENDENCE	EFFECTS	SLANG NAMES
Yes	Yes	Yes	Euphoria, relaxation, lowered inhibitions	Booze, juice, hooch
Yes	Yes	Yes	Temporary euphoria and sense of well-being	H, horse, shit, scag, junk, smack, hard stuff, Harry, snow, caballo, Doojee, boy, hairy, joy powder, dope, schmeek, thing
Yes	Yes	Yes	Euphoria, drowsiness and stupor, sense of unreality	Op
Yes	Yes	Yes	Relieves pain, causes drowsiness, induces sleep	M, dreamer, white stuff, hard stuff, morpho, unkie, Miss Emma, monkey, cube, morf, tab, emsel, hocus, morphie, melter
Yes	Yes	Yes	Same as morphine	Schoolboy
Yes	Yes	Yes	Same as opiúm	Dolly, doll
No	No	Possible	Euphoria, relaxation, sociability	Weed, grass, smoke, pot, straw, Texas tea, jive, matah, splim, Acapulco Gold, Bhang, boo, bush, butter flower, muggles, hemp, griffo, Indian hay, loco weed, herb, J, mu, giggles-smoke, love, Mary Warner, Mary Jane, love weed, joints, reefers, sativa, roach, Greta, mezz

DRUG	CHAPTER	LEGITIMATE MEDICAL USES	METHODS OF USE	TYPICAL DOSE	DURATION OF ACTION
Hallucinogens (too numerous to list)	6	Experimental use in treatment of alcoholism and mental illness	Swallowed	Varies, depending on drug	2–12 hours, depending on drug and dosage
Barbiturates (depressants/ sedative hypnotics)	3	To induce sedation and anesthesia, and to prevent convulsions	Swallowed in pill form or injected	50–100 mg	4 hours
Amphetamines (stimulants)	7	Treatment of fatigue, depression, narcolepsy, hyperactivity, and obesity	Swallowed in pill form or injected into the vein	5–30 mg	4–12 hours
Cocaine (stimulant)	7	Local anesthetic	Sniffed or injected	Variable	20 minutes or longer
Tranquilizers (mild depressants/sedatives)	3	Relief of anxiety and tension. Treatment of alcoholism, psychological disorders, and vomiting	Swallowed	5–10 mg	4–6 hours
Inhalants (solvents)	3	None	Sniffed	Variable	1–2 hours

POTENTIAL FOR DEVELOPMENT OF TOLERANCE	PHYSICAL DEPENDENCE	PSYCHOLOGICAL DEPENDENCE	EFFECTS	SLANG NAMES
Possible with continued use	No	Minimal	Range from mild states of euphoria and intensified sensory perception to wild illusions and hallucinations	Too numerous to list
Yes	Yes	Yes	Relaxation, euphoria, drowsiness, and sleep	Yellows, yellow jackets, nimby, nimbles, reds, pinks, red birds, red devils, seggy, seccy, pink ladies, blues, blue birds, blue devils, blue heavens, double trouble, tooies, Christmas trees, phennies, barbs
Yes	Perhaps	Yes	Increased wakefulness, alertness, euphoria, loss of appetite	Speed, uppers, pep pills, bennies, wake-ups, eye-openers, lid-poppers, copilots, truck drivers, peaches, roses, hearts, cartwheels
Yes	No	Yes	Increased alertness, loss of appetite, euphoria	Coke, snow, the leaf, C, cecil, flake, speedball (when mixed with heroin), girl, happy dust, joy powder, white girl, gold dust, Corine, dynamite, Bernies, Burese, gin, Bernice, stardust, Carrie, Cholly, heaven dust, paradise
Yes	Perhaps	Minimal	Relief of anxiety and tension	
Yes	No	Perhaps	Euphoria, hallucinations	

particular group or subculture. However, direct or indirect pressure to use drugs is sometimes exerted by one's peers and the nonuser may be ridiculed or even excluded from the group's activities.

It should also be noted that a high proportion of drug abusers, although certainly not all, suffer from personality disturbances and, to a certain extent, drug abuse may be related to this fact.[6]

Addiction: Tolerance and Dependence

Many drugs, when used for the first time, can produce extremely unpleasant effects. The first time a person tries heroin, for example, he or she may actually become physically ill. Likewise, the initial use of LSD can be a very frightening experience. In the case of such drugs, the role of one's peers becomes extremely important in maintaining the new user's interest in the drug. Friends are likely to try to convince the new drug user that the adverse effects of the drug are to be expected at first, that they happen to everyone, and that the "best" is yet to come.

The continued use of a drug having a high addiction potential eventually gives rise to certain physiological processes which play an important role in maintaining drug use. These are the development of tolerance and physical dependence. *Tolerance* refers to a condition in which increased quantities of the drug are required to produce the desired effects. *Physical dependence* is said to be present when discontinuation of the drug results in a reaction by the body called the *withdrawal* or *abstinence syndrome*. This syndrome, which varies in severity according to the degree of the addiction, is a result of the body's having developed an actual physical need for the drug in order to maintain normal functioning. *Psychological dependence,* which usually accompanies physical dependence, refers to both the need to avoid the symptoms of the withdrawal syndrome and the need to maintain the sense of "well-being" associated with continued use of the drug.

Addiction occurs when the user becomes both physically and psychologically dependent upon the effects of the drug. A person who is addicted to a drug may exhibit one or more of the following behaviors:

1. A pronounced desire to take the drug after it has not been taken for a while.
2. A reorientation of one's life so that obtaining the drug becomes a major activity.
3. A high likelihood of relapse after discontinuation of use and subsequent withdrawal.

In terms of these criteria, the drugs having the highest *addiction potential* are alcohol, opiates, barbiturates and other sedatives, and certain tranquilizers. Addiction potential is lower or not known to be present for stimulants, marijuana, the hallucinogens, and the inhalants and solvents.

How Drugs Are Administered

In order for a drug to produce its effects it must be introduced into the user's body. There are a variety of ways of accomplishing this, depending upon the drug. Heroin, for instance, may be injected directly into a vein, under the skin, or into a muscle, or it may be sniffed, smoked, or ingested orally. Amphetamines may either be taken orally or injected. Marijuana may be smoked or eaten, and its active ingredient, THC, may be injected. Naturally, the method of administration depends upon the form in which the drug is available to the user. Table 1.1 lists the most common methods of administration for each drug.

One important fact to remember is that the method used to administer a drug will have a definite influence on the effects that it produces. For example, a dose of heroin injected directly into the vein will have a much more rapid onset of response than the same dose injected under the skin or into the muscle. But regardless of how or where the drug is injected, this method will always produce more rapid effects than oral administration. When a drug is taken orally, additional time is required for its active substance to enter the bloodstream so that it can be transported to the brain, where its effects are produced. In order for a drug that is injested orally to reach the bloodstream, it must first be dissolved in the stomach fluid and then, depending on the particular drug, be absorbed through the stomach wall or transported to the intestine, where it is absorbed through the intestinal wall into the bloodstream. When a drug is injected directly into the muscle, it is absorbed much more rapidly than when it is taken orally, but regardless of the method used, the drug must always be absorbed into the bloodstream before its effects can be felt.

Another factor which may determine the ultimate effect of an orally administered drug is the *amount* of the drug that is actually absorbed into the tissues. This may depend upon (1) the dissolvability of the drug; and (2) the effects of the digestive juices on its active ingredient(s). Generally speaking, drugs that are taken orally have the slowest onset of action.

The inhalation of a drug may result in a more rapid onset of action, depending on the size of the particles of the drug being inhaled. However, inhalation is less efficient than injection because much of the drug's active ingredient may be lost and hence it fails to reach the lungs.

Of all the modes of administration described above, injection carries the greatest risk because foreign substances may be introduced into the body, causing infection or other complications. Injection also carries the risk of damaging a nerve.

How Drugs Produce Their Effects

Drug effects are produced in the central nervous system (C.N.S.). Thus, a drug can only be effective to the extent to which it is present in the brain. The sooner it reaches the C.N.S., the sooner its effects will be felt; the longer it remains there, the longer its duration of action. (How long a psychologically active drug remains in the body has no effect on the duration of its effects. Rather, it is how long the drug remains in the C.N.S. that determines the length of its action.)

Once in the brain, a drug only acts at certain locations. These locations vary depending on the drug. This in part accounts for the different effects of different drugs, because each part of the brain has different functions. Almost all psychoactive drugs act at more than one location in the brain.

The brain itself is composed of billions of nerve cells which carry information from one part of the brain to another, much like a giant switchboard. Messages enter the brain, carrying information about changes in both the external and internal environment. Once this information enters the brain it is carried along nerve pathways to specific centers where the information is processed. Finally, messages are sent from the appropriate brain centers to initiate changes in the body. This entire process may take place in only a fraction of a second.

Carrying the switchboard analogy one step farther, the many nerve cells, or *neurons,* which make up the brain might be thought of as wires or circuits along which information is carried. Each of these neurons connects to one or more other neurons. The point at which two neurons connect is called the *synapse*. The actual transmission of information across the space between nerve cells at the synapse (or *synaptic cleft*) is carried out by chemical substances called *neurotransmitters*. The neurotransmitters are released by one cell, in which they have been stored, flow across the dividing space, and stimulate the adjoining cell or cells, which then continue to carry the message. After this process has been completed, *enzymes* present at the synapse neutralize the transmitter substance so that the synapse is again ready to carry a new message. Any interference with this process of transmission will result in a modification of the information received by the second cell. For example, if the active chemical substance present in a drug increases the amount of neurotransmitter substance released at the synapse by the presynaptic cell, the postsynaptic cell will become "overexcited." If the drug decreases the amount of neurotransmitter substance released, the postsynaptic cell will be understimulated.

A drug may also act by interfering with the release of enzymes. If the correct amount of enzyme is not released after the chemical transmitter has been released at the synapse, the transmitter may remain active for a longer period of time than would normally be the case. Other drugs may affect different enzymes which are involved in building neurotransmitters. Should this occur, the amount of neurotransmitter produced will be decreased, and the normal synaptic transmission will be lessened.

What is important to remember is that although all psychoactive drugs affect the process of synaptic transmission, different drugs may affect different neurotransmitter substances in different ways. Generally speaking, sedative (or sleep-inducing) drugs *depress* synaptic activity in certain brain centers, whereas stimulant drugs *increase* the rate of activity at synapses. A good example of the latter is the action of cocaine, a strong stimulant which produces its excitatory effects by increasing the amount of *norepinephrine* (a neurotransmitter substance) present at the synapse. This increase occurs because of cocaine's interference with the "re-uptake" of norepinephrine after its initial release, thus leaving norepinephrine capable of continued action for an extended period of time.

The Nervous System

We have discussed how the effects of psychoactive drugs are related to their interference with the transmission of information between nerve cells. However, to discuss these effects in greater detail it would be necessary to devote an entire chapter to the anatomy of the human nervous system. Thus, we will limit our discussion to *functional levels* within the nervous system as well as to the major divisions of the nervous system.

At the lowest level of the nervous system is the *spinal cord*. The spinal cord carries information to and from the brain and brain stem on the one hand, and to the rest of the body on the other. It also contains centers controlling simple reflexes, such as the sudden withdrawal of a finger when one touches a hot stove.

The *brain stem* connects the spinal cord and the brain. The brain stem is made up of the *medulla*, the *pons*, and the *midbrain*. The most important of these three structures in determining the effects of a given drug is the medulla. This structure contains the controlling centers for many bodily activities necessary for life, including breathing, heartbeat, and blood pressure. Thus, it has been called the "vital center of the brain."[7] If these centers are sufficiently depressed—say, by a large dose of a depressant drug—death may occur. Passing through the medulla is a diffuse structure called the *reticular formation*. This structure, part of which is referred to as the *reticular activating system*, or *RAS*, plays an important role in maintaining alertness and in regulating sleep and wakefulness. Many drugs that are used as sedatives or that have sedative side effects, such as the barbiturates, depress this center, thus decreasing the amount of information that can be carried by it to the brain. Some stimulant drugs, such as the amphetamines, increase the activity of the RAS, thus increasing the level of alertness. Likewise, some of the excitatory effects produced by hallucinogenic drugs such as LSD may be related to the fact that these drugs increase the responsiveness of the RAS to external stimulation.

The *cerebellum*, which is located behind the midbrain, is concerned with coordination of muscular activity. Depression of the activity of the cerebellum by such drugs as alcohol may explain the lack of coordination observed in an intoxicated person.

The *forebrain* consists of the thalamus, the hypothalamus, the basal ganglia, the limbic system, and the cerebrum. Only some of these structures will be discussed here.

The *thalamus* is a way station for nerve fibers coming to the cerebral cortex from the brain stem and spinal cord. Below the thalamus is the *hypothalamus*. This small structure contains centers for the regulation of the blood levels of many important body chemicals, as well as centers for controlling temperature, hunger, water balance and thirst, and sex. Centers which are involved in the regulation of emotion and mood are also located here. The hypothalamus is part of the *limbic system*—which regulates emotional behavior—and it is here that some tranquilizers are believed to act.

The *cerebral cortex,* the ''highest'' level of the brain, is composed of two hemispheres. It is responsible for sensory, motor, and association functions. In general, it is the first part of the brain to be affected by a psychoactive drug, especially the depressants. Because it has inhibiting effects on the lower centers of the brain, depression of the cerebral cortex results in less restraint being applied to these lower centers. Thus, some depressants, such as alcohol and the barbiturates, at first appear to have a stimulatory effect on the user. Increased ingestion of depressants eventually results in depression of the activity of lower centers, first interfering with coordination, and finally with respiration. This pattern of successive depression of the various levels of the nervous system will be examined in the next chapter, which discusses the effects of alcohol.

Finally, there is the *autonomic nervous system*. This system, composed of structures outside the central nervous system, contains two divisions or subsystems which play an important role in producing the effects we see in many drug-induced states. The *sympathetic system* stimulates or increases the rate of action of many internal organs, glands, and blood vessels. Thus, if stimulated, we see a pattern of increased heart rate, fast and shallow breathing, and sweating. The amphetamines and cocaine produce physical effects that are highly similar to those produced by stimulation of the sympathetic system. The *parasympathetic system* generally has opposite effects when stimulated, including decreased heart rate and slower and deeper breathing.

Drugs Affect People Differently

A question that frequently arises when drugs are discussed is why two different people sometimes respond to the same drug in such different ways. The answer is simply that no two people are in exactly the same physical, mental, and emotional condition when the drug is taken. For instance, a person's body weight will have a definite influence on the level of intoxication produced by a given amount of alcohol. Likewise, the amount of food present in the stomach at the time the drug is taken may be an important factor. Previous experience with the drug is also an influential factor—the user may have developed a degree of tolerance to the effects of the drug or, because of prior experience, may be more knowledgeable about the drug's effects and thus respond to it differently. In addition, whether or not other drugs have been used recently may be a factor in determining how a person will respond to a particular drug; the psychological and emotional state of the user is also important. Even the circumstances under which the drug is taken may influence the effects the user experiences. For example, a person who takes a hallucinogenic drug in the company of friends may have a much more pleasant experience than one who takes the same drug in a strange or unfamiliar setting. Therefore, it is extremely difficult to predict the effects that a particular drug will produce. To further complicate this problem the user of illicit drugs seldom knows the purity or the actual dose level of the drug he or she is taking.

Notes

1. O. S. Ray, *Drugs, Society, and Human Behavior* (St. Louis: Mosby, 1972), p. 79.
2. J. A. Cimino et al, ''Narcotic Addiction in the United States: A Nationwide Survey,'' *Contemporary Drug Problems* 2 (1973): pp. 401–415.
3. J. J. Platt, W. C. Scura, and A. R. Hoffman, ''Heroin Addiction Incidence Among Youthful Offenders, 1968–1972,'' *Journal of Community Psychology* 1 (1973): pp. 408–411.
4. J. H. Jaffe, ''Drug Addiction and Drug Abuse,'' in L. S. Goodman and A. Gilman, eds., *The Pharmacological Basis of Therapeutics*, 4th ed. (New York: Macmillan, 1970), p. 276.
5. J. C. Ball, ''Marijuana Smoking and the Onset of Heroin Abuse,'' in J. O. Cole and J. R. Wittenborn, eds., *Drug Abuse: Social and Psychopharmacological Aspects* (Springfield, Ill.: Thomas, 1966), p. 126.
6. J. J. Platt and C. Labate, *Heroin Addiction: Theory, Research, and Treatment* (New York: Wiley-Interscience, 1976), p. 154.
7. C. T. Morgan, *Physiological Psychology*, 3rd ed. (New York: McGraw-Hill, 1965), p. 39.

Selected Bibliography

Bourne, P. G., ed. *Addiction*. New York: Academic Press, 1974.

Hofmann, F. G. *A Handbook on Drug and Alcohol Abuse*. New York: Oxford, 1975.

Leavitt, F. *Drugs and Behavior*. Philadelphia: Saunders, 1974.

President's Commission on Law Enforcement and Administration of Justice. *Task Force Report: Narcotics and Drug Abuse*. Washington, D.C.: U.S. Government Printing Office, 1967.

Ray, O. S. *Drugs, Society, and Human Behavior*. St. Louis: Mosby, 1972.

Chapter 2

Depressants: Alcohol

A drug user who buys heroin or some other drug on the street has no way of determining the quality of the drug in advance. In fact, there is no guarantee that the user will get what he or she expects. On the one hand, the strength of the dose may be sufficient to make the user violently ill, but on the other hand, it may be so weak as to fail to produce any effect at all. "Street heroin," for example, may either be practically pure or it may be so significantly "cut" (mixed) with another substance—ranging all the way from sugar to rat poison—that the actual heroin content in the dose is negligible.

With alcohol, however, this is not the case. The buyer gets exactly what is paid for—but just what does the user get?

Alcohol and Its Effects

Alcohol is available in many forms, but when we speak of the alcohol contained in an intoxicating beverage, the word refers to ethanol or ethyl alcohol. This alcohol is initially obtained through the fermentation of sugars and starches. However, to produce intoxicating beverages with a higher alcoholic content than that of beer or wine—say, for example, rum, whiskey, or gin—a process of distillation must also be undertaken.

In distillation, a liquid mixture is vaporized and the components of the vapor are collected by differential cooling during condensation. In distilling a previously fermented solution containing a low concentration of alcohol in order to produce a beverage with a greater alcoholic content, heat must be applied to the solution until the alcohol, which has a lower boiling point than water, is changed to a vapor. This vapor is then collected and condensed into a liquid form again, resulting in a new beverage having a higher alcoholic *proof* (one-half of the proof equals the percent of actual alcohol content—in other words, 86 proof means that the alcohol is 43 percent of the total liquid content).

Regardless of the alcoholic content of an intoxicating beverage, once it is ingested it travels to the stomach and small intestine, where it is absorbed, and then it is distributed generally throughout the body. The rate at which the alcohol is absorbed into the tissues may be affected by a number of factors:

1. *Alcohol concentration.* The greater the alcohol concentration of the beverage—up to a maximum of about 40 percent (80 proof)—the more rapidly the alcohol is absorbed and the higher are the resulting peak blood-alcohol concentrations. The highest blood-alcohol levels are produced by undiluted distilled spirits, and the lowest by beers.
2. *Other chemicals in the beverage.* The greater the amount of nonalcoholic chemicals in the beverage, the more slowly the alcohol is absorbed. This explains why the alcohol contained in distilled spirits—especially vodka and gin—is absorbed more rapidly than that found in table wines and beers.
3. *Presence of food in the stomach.* The ingestion of food along with drinking has a notable effect on the amount of alcohol that enters the bloodstream. Thus, when alcoholic beverages are taken with a substantial meal, peak blood-alcohol concentrations may be reduced by as much as 50 percent.
4. *Speed of drinking.* The more rapidly the beverage is ingested, the higher will be the resulting peak blood-alcohol concentrations. Thus, these levels are lower when the beverage is sipped or taken in divided amounts than when it is gulped or taken in a single dose.
5. *Emptying time of the stomach.* In a number of clinical conditions, such as that marked by the "dumping syndrome," the stomach empties more rapidly than is normal, and alcohol seems to be absorbed more quickly. Emptying time may be either slowed down or accelerated by fear, anger, stress, nausea, or the condition of the stomach tissues.
6. *Body weight.* The greater the body weight of an individual, the lower will be the blood-alcohol concentration resulting from ingestion of a standard amount of alcohol. The blood-alcohol level of a 180-lb. person consuming four ounces of distilled spirits, for example, will be substantially lower than that of a 130-lb. person consuming the same amount in the same length of time.[1]

Regardless of the rate of absorption, however, once certain blood levels are reached, a number of effects can be expected:

1. At 0.05 percent the individual is usually euphoric; alertness is in fact already lowered at this point. To reach this level a 150-lb. person would probably need to drink two beers or two glasses of wine within a period of one hour.
2. At 0.10 percent the drinker is less inhibited; the person starts to throw caution to the wind and reaction time is noticeably lengthened.
3. At 0.20 percent the individual may become dizzy; visual-motor coordination is significantly depressed. (Many people believe alcohol to be a stimulant because it breaks down the drinker's normal inhibitions but, in reality, it is a general anesthetic, capable of depressing central nervous system functioning.) A 150-lb. person would have to consume approximately three glasses of beer or wine within a period of one hour to reach the 0.20 percent alcohol blood level.
4. At 0.25 percent the individual may begin to stagger and slur words; visual-motor coordination is quite markedly impaired at this point.
5. At 0.30 percent the person is in a semistuporous state.
6. At 0.40 percent the alcohol blood level is lethal (this statistic applies to 50 percent of the population).

Alcohol then not only leads to euphoria but if consumed in sufficiently large quantities can cause delayed reaction time, impaired visual-motor coordination, sedation, anesthesia, and even death. These reactions have been experienced by people down through the ages. The users and abusers of alcohol are by no means new to the "drug scene." In fact, until quite recently, the use of alcohol virtually dominated the drug scene. As a matter of fact, although other drugs are being widely experimented with now, alcohol is again a growing problem, particularly among teenagers.

How Alcohol Produces Its Effects

As noted above, many people are under the mistaken impression that alcohol is a stimulant because drinking small-to-moderate amounts of the drug often produces euphoric effects, accompanied by an increase in relaxation and a heightened sense of well-being and self-confidence. But alcohol is actually a very potent depressant whose apparent stimulatory effects are the result of the depression of or interference with those parts of the brain that inhibit or regulate behavior. As anyone who has ever watched another person drink to excess knows, the effects of alcohol are progressive. As the drinker ingests more and more alcohol, mental and physical functioning becomes increasingly impaired. This is due to the progressive interference by alcohol with brain functioning. First, the highest centers of the brain—those dealing with prior learning—are depressed, producing the seeming euphoria described above; then successively lower centers are depressed resulting in erratic changes of mood, followed by loss of motor control, general impairment of functioning, and, finally, sleep. With ingestion of very large doses of alcohol, anesthesia, coma, and eventually death may occur. When death occurs, the immediate cause is in most cases the result of depression of the respiratory centers in the brain.

To produce its effects, alcohol must reach the bloodstream and eventually make its way to the brain. Although some alcohol reaches the bloodstream by being absorbed through the wall of the stomach, most of it (about 80 percent) enters the blood from the upper intestine. Because the presence of food in the stomach decreases alcohol absorption, absorption will be slower for the individual who has eaten before drinking than for the individual who drinks on an empty stomach.

Once alcohol reaches the brain, it rapidly produces the depressant effects noted above, starting with the highest centers of the brain. The specific way in which alcohol interferes with brain functioning at any level is by depressing transmission of impulses at the synaptic junctions between nerve cells.

Before alcohol can leave the body, most of it (over 90 percent) must be converted, or metabolized, by the liver to carbon dioxide and water. Unlike other drugs, however, the rate at which alcohol is converted is not proportionate to the amount of alcohol in the blood, but occurs at a steady rate equal to approximately the amount contained in one ounce of liquor being converted each hour. Because there is no practical way to increase this rate of conversion, the drinker will remain intoxicated for approximately as many hours as he or she has imbibed ounces of liquor.

The drinker experiences a number of physiological changes. First, there is an increase in the flow of blood to the stomach, which leads to an increase in the flow of digestive secretions. Second, alcohol causes the blood vessels near the skin to dilate, resulting in a flushed appearance accompanied by a feeling of increased warmth. Many people believe that drinking alcohol is a good way to stay warm in cold weather, but this notion is false because drinking actually causes a *loss* of body heat. The feeling of warmth experienced by the drinker is merely the result of the dilation of blood vessels. The fact is that large amounts of alcohol actually *lower* body temperature by directly depressing the temperature-regulating center of the brain. Third, drinking causes an increased secretion of urine by the kidneys. And, finally, it can lead to vomiting, although usually not until the blood-alcohol level has reached about 0.12 percent; this may serve a life-saving purpose because by emptying the drinker's stomach, it helps prevent further absorption of the alcohol. The long-term consequences of alcoholism will be described later in the chapter.

The Abuse of Alcohol

It is difficult to know exactly how long alcohol has been in use, but it has been estimated that perhaps as early as 8000 B.C. people were using (and possibly even abusing) alcoholic beverages. In 4000 B.C. wine and beer were used in Egypt. And the Bible is replete with accounts of alcohol use. Although the moderate use of alcohol was considered to be an acceptable practice during these early periods, drunkenness was often publicly denounced. One of the earliest documents encouraging temperance was written in Egypt some 3,000 years ago, under the title *Wisdom of Ani*. "Take not upon thyself to drink a jug of beer," it advocated. "Thou speakest, and an unintelligible utterance issueth from thy mouth. If thou fallest down and thy limbs break, there is none to hold out a hand to thee. Thy companions in drink stand up and say 'Away with this sot.' And thou are like a little child."[2]

Today, drinking is a highly acceptable and widely abused practice. If there has been a change in attitude since the days of antiquity, it is probably for the worse. Partly in response to the $350-million advertising campaign waged by the alcoholic beverage industry each year, the equivalent of close to ten quarts of pure alcohol per adult is being consumed annually in the United States. Regardless of whether people drink as a result of provocative ads that pair yachts and expensive wines or light beers and sports, or because of such socially acceptable occasions as drinking business lunches or the evening cocktail hour, the fact remains that today close to 80 percent of all urban adults report having taken an alcoholic beverage at one time or another.

Within this group of urban drinkers, and the reported 50 percent of the rural population who have used alcoholic beverages, a large number *abuse* alcohol on a regular basis. In fact, it is estimated that there are over nine million alcoholics in the United States alone.

The reported waste of time and money, not to mention the personal suffering that results from alcohol abuse is staggering. The federal government estimates that between $275 and $550 million are lost each year as a result of alcoholism among civil service employees. Losses in industry owing to alcoholism have been computed at $10 billion per year. The personal suffering of alcoholics, as well as that of their families and friends, is one that cannot be measured in terms of dollars.

Why people drink is a question for which one can quickly and logically formulate a number of answers. In addition to the euphoria it brings and the social function it serves, alcohol is also used to relieve tension and anxiety, to boost a sagging ego, to dull the inner pain of depression, to release inhibitions, or to cause oblivion (blackout) so that the drinker does not have to remember or feel responsible for repressed desires.

What is more difficult to understand is why some people who drink become alcoholics and others do not. (For our purposes, an alcoholic is a person who uses alcohol to the extent that it interferes with the ability to function normally on a day-to-day basis.) Is the answer related to some physiological, pharmacological, or pathological appetite for alcohol? Or is there some common psychological characteristic or personality trait that is shared by all alcoholics? The problem of identifying the potential alcoholic is a very complex, and often disputed, one. The fact is that this issue is far too intricate to be discussed at any length in a single chapter, much less a few paragraphs. However, in order to gain some insight into the problem, it might be useful to understand how alcoholism progresses.

A person typically passes through a number of fairly well defined stages on the way to becoming an alcoholic. Although it is true that some alcoholics seem to remain at one stage throughout their entire lives, whereas others progress rapidly from one stage to another, perhaps even skipping some of them in the process, they all encounter many of the same problems along the way. Listed below are nine stages of alcoholism; these stages are valuable because they offer some important clues about the behavior patterns of individuals who eventually develop serious drinking problems or who become alcoholics.

Stage One: The Novice. Most people never progress beyond this initial stage. Drinks are usually taken in moderation and then only at social functions. On occasion, the individual at this stage may drink to excess, experiencing a "hangover" the following morning.

Stage Two: Onset of Heavy Drinking and Blackouts. At this stage the individual begins to drink heavily at bars or at parties and often has trouble later remembering what happened during a drinking bout.

Stage Three: Required Additional Drinking. At this stage the person finds it increasingly difficult to "get high" and may become self-conscious about his or her drinking. Often the person drinks before going to a party or social event in order to conceal from others the amount of liquor that he or she needs to become intoxicated.

Stage Four: Early Signs of Control Loss. The individual at this stage can no longer control how much he or she will drink on a given occasion. Such a person can, however, control when the first drink will be taken.

Stage Five: Excuse Drinking. At this stage the drinker may abstain from using alcohol for long periods of time (possibly even months) in an attempt to prove that he or she does not *need* to drink. However, once the drinking behavior is resumed, the individual drinks heavily, which naturally produces feelings of guilt. In order to assuage this guilt, the drinker invents excuses for drinking, claiming, for example, that he or she is celebrating some occasion or has been working too hard and needs a few drinks in order to relax.

Stage Six: Drinking Alone. At this stage alcohol has become the individual's best friend. The drinker now drinks alone so that excuses for drinking are no longer necessary. The person at this stage gradually moves into a self-imposed dreamworld which allows him or her to go on drinking without having to face what is actually happening.

Stage Seven: Hostile, Sensitive Drinker. At this stage the drinker becomes somewhat antisocial. The drinker may provoke unnecessary fights with friends and relatives, and begin abusing others—both verbally and physically—without experiencing any apparent remorse.

Stage Eight: Extended Drinking and "Benders." At this stage, the person drinks in the morning to "treat" the hangover from the previous evening's drinking bout. The drinker also begins going on "benders," that is, extended bouts of drinking. During this period the drinker has lost most if not all concern for personal welfare as well as that of others.

Stage Nine: "Hitting Bottom." In this final stage, the alcoholic has given up everything for drink. The drinker may remain at this point until continued drinking finally results in death—either directly or indirectly—or he or she may seek treatment. Unfortunately, because the drinker or the drinker's family failed to recognize the problem at an earlier state, by this point the drinker may have lost everything he or she had prior to becoming an alcoholic. Had the drinker sought treatment at an earlier stage, much human misery might have been avoided.

Alcoholism and Physical Health

Alcohol taken in small-to-moderate amounts does not have any serious physical effects. However, the continued use of large amounts of alcohol over a long period of time may have disastrous effects on all aspects of mental and physical functioning. Among the adverse effects of alcoholism on the body are: (1) *cirrhosis of the liver,* which occurs in some 8 percent of all chronic alcoholics and involves the destruction of liver cells and their replacement by fatty tissue; (2) *malnutrition* and *vitamin deficiencies,* which result from decreased food intake and contribute to the development of cirrhosis of the liver; (3) *interference with the digestive process,* including decrease of stomach digestive activities, irritation of the colon and pancreas, and constipation or diarrhea; (4) *decrease or absence of sexual functioning;* and (5) *increased susceptibility to infections and other diseases* due to improper nutrition, vitamin deficiences, and generally poor physical condition.

The fact that regular intake of large amounts of alcohol results in the development of alcohol dependence means that when its use is discontinued, the symptoms of the withdrawal syndrome will appear. In the case of alcohol, this set of symptoms is known as *delirium tremens* (or the d.t.'s) and may involve hallucinations, exhaustion, confusion, insomnia, tremors, and agitation. In extremely severe cases, withholding alcohol from an alcoholic may result in convulsions and even death.

There are many different types of treatment and rehabilitation programs available to the alcoholic. For a more detailed discussion of the various therapeutic approaches, see Chapter 8.

The Use of Alcohol and the Criminal Justice System

Alcohol use has almost always been an issue of major importance for local, state, and federal criminal justice agencies in the United States. The primary concerns of these agencies center around the following issues regarding alcohol consumption:

1. Regulation
2. Law enforcement agents as primary care personnel with alcoholics
3. Driving under the influence of alcohol.

Regulation

In China, as early as 1100 B.C. laws were being imposed in connection with the sale and consumption of alcoholic beverages. Attempts in Europe to limit alcohol use spanned from the fourteenth to the early part of the twentieth century. In England we find typical examples of legal restrictions of alcohol use. In the sixth, fourteenth, and nineteenth centuries, religious edicts and civil laws were enacted in an effort to temper the use of alcohol. What is surprising, by contemporary standards, is that despite the emotional outcries of the day against alcohol's evil influences (''decent women . . .'' and ''young prostitutes from twelve to fourteen years of age . . . were being charged with being drunk and disorderly''), many of the laws designed to temper alcohol abuse were relatively mild. In 1839, for example, the primary sections of the public drunkenness act initiated the policy of weekend closing times for establishments selling alcoholic beverages and established a legal drinking age—one had to be at least sixteen years of age.

In the English colonies the regulations imposed on alcohol users and abusers are interesting in their own right. Connecticut (1659) fined a person $5 for becoming drunk ''in his own home.'' Virginia (in 1664 and again in 1760) passed laws prohibiting ministers from ''drinking to excess'' and ''inciting riot.'' Georgia (1755), on the other hand, would not issue a liquor license to ''any tradesman who was capable of making his livelihood by honest labor.''

Once the colonies gained their independence they became free to enact new federal and state laws to regulate alcoholic beverages on their own. And that they did. In 1791 a federal excise tax was placed on whiskey; in 1834 a congressional law was passed prohibiting the sale of alcoholic beverages to Indians; and in 1851 Maine enacted the first prohibition law.

Prohibition periods on local, state, and federal levels are part of the American tradition. Beginning with Maine's law, a series of regulations would be passed and repealed until December 5, 1933, when the Twenty-first Amendment was ratified by thirty-six states, thus ending the ''Great Prohibition.''

Clearly, then, there was never any firm or lasting stand taken against the use of alcohol. This possibly stems not only from the fact that alcoholic beverages had accepted uses in religious ceremonies and unwritten medical prescriptions, but also because its social use—and the clubs and saloons that grew up around it—had become part of the American way of life. In 1889, for instance, some leading community members described the saloon in a quite favorable light.

> It is a center of learning, books, papers, and lecture hall to them [workingmen]. It is the clearinghouse for common intelligence, the place where their philosophy of life is worked out, and their political and social beliefs take their beginnings.[3]

Furthermore, the question of the effectiveness of prohibition and stringent regulation of alcohol use is questionable. Dry counties, established in the early twentieth century, led to an increase rather than a decrease in per capita alcohol consumption. Prohibition's success in the 1920s was also disputable. Although alcohol consumption, cirrhosis of the liver, and alcohol-related death rates did initially drop, they rose again during the later years of prohibition to almost preprohibition rates. Prohibition was indeed a qualified failure.

Today, wine, beer, and liquor regulation enforcement by criminal justice agencies involves violations arising from sale of alcoholic beverages to minors, diluting alcohol by bars and restaurants, alcoholic beverage smuggling and other related tax evasion activities, and enforcement of "blue laws" and closing times of alcoholic beverage outlets (stores, bars, and so forth).

However, enforcement agencies today are primarily concerned with the problem of handling intoxicated persons, particularly those cited for driving under the influence of alcohol. The Federal Bureau of Investigation reports that one out of every three arrests involves alcohol abuse; approximately two million arrests for the offense of public drunkenness are made by police agencies annually in the United States; practically one-half of all fatal accidents today involve an alcoholic; over 90 percent of short-term prisoners are confined because of their contact with alcohol; the suicide rate for alcoholics compared to nonalcoholics is 58 to 1.

Handling the Intoxicated Person or the Alcoholic

Even in those few areas of the country where there are no specific laws dealing with drunkenness, inebriates are still often locked up under other charges such as vagrancy, loitering, and disorderly conduct. Maximum penalties for drunkenness range from five days to six months; for habitual drunkenness, some states even have statutes under which a person can be imprisoned for up to two years.

In addition to the estimated yearly cost of $100 million to handle drunken individuals, the President's Crime Commission points out the generally unfortunate results of classifying drunkenness as a crime problem.

> The criminal justice system appears ineffective to deter drunkenness or to meet the problems of the chronic alcoholic offender. What the system does accomplish is to remove the drunk from public view, detoxify him, and provide him with food, shelter, emergency medical service, and a brief period of forced sobriety. As presently constituted, the system is not in a position to meet his underlying medical and social problems . . . Drunkenness should not itself be a criminal offense.[4]

Until the laws are changed the peace officer will continue to be responsible for handling inebriates. Therefore, to enable police, sheriffs, and correction officers to deal with drunken individuals as optimally as possible, information must be available to help them undertake this task. In response to this need the Smithers Foundation published a handbook on the subject, *Alcohol and Alcoholism: A Police Handbook*. The following is an excerpt from the section titled "Handling the Intoxicated Person or Alcoholic."

> In handling the "drunk" or alcoholic in your course of duty as a police officer, you will encounter many different problems. Knowing how to handle these could, in some cases, mean the difference between life and death. Your very first problem will be to determine the extent of drunkenness. You must decide whether

the person is in such a state as to be capable of hurting himself or others. If he does seem potentially dangerous, then he must be taken into custody, or at least protected.

With the sleepy, depressed type, you must be especially careful. He may appear quite capable of sleeping off his current state of intoxication. But he may have downed a pint or more of whiskey, or some such drink, just before you arrested him—in which case, he will get more and more intoxicated in the following hour or two. If left alone in a cell and not watched, he could die from absorption of extra alcohol during that time. So your second problem involves your ability to recognize some of the common danger signs and complications of severe intoxication.

Possible Complications:

Coma—Initially the victim is drowsy, very sad, and sick. He may be aggressive when disturbed. Later he may develop some definite physical signs, such as skin pallor. Looking at him you will see his eyes crossed or pointing out. He may complain of ringing in his ears, numbness "all over," and seeing double. His pulse becomes rapid, the eye pupils—tiny in the first stage—now become very large. Later he goes into increasing stupor, from which it is difficult to arouse him, and he may die of two things:

Shock—signs are paleness, sweating, clammy skin, fainting, and weak pulse;

Total anesthesia of the brain—this could happen within two or three hours of first seeing a drunken person.

Convulsions—These are a possibly frightening, possibly dangerous development of the hangover stage. The immediate dangers are that the victim may fall and hurt himself or that his airway may become blocked, so-called swallowing of the tongue. The general danger is that the convulsion may indicate a very serious medical condition. The best treatment is to lay the convulsive patient on his back, if possible, loosen any tight clothing, and put something soft, such as a rolled-up shirttail, in the corner of his mouth. This will prevent him from biting his tongue and will give him an airway. After administering first aid a physician should be called, and the person should be watched until medical advice is obtained.

Alcoholic Hallucinosis—This lasts from minutes to days. The victim sees and hears things that are not really there. He is convinced that they are there, and they may be vivid, frightening, and terrifying. Sometimes he may have delusions (feeling perhaps someone is after his life). Apart from these abnormalities, however, he is rational, can talk, and knows who you are and what time of day it is. He doesn't usually have a fast pulse, fever, or tremor, and is not sweating, pale, or flushed. In fact, he looks all right, but "sees things."

Delirium Tremens—This is a serious possible complication of the hangover stage. The person suffering from delirium tremens is out of contact with his surroundings and does not know what is going on though there may be clear periods. You may wear a uniform, but he will not necessarily recognize this or realize what it means. He may not know where he is, what time of day or what month it is, or even what nationality he is. He doesn't "know" anything! He often has some fever, is flushed, has a rapid pulse and intense tremor. In addition, he has the typical disturbing hallucinations and suffers from insomnia and great exhaustion. Usually the condition lasts from two to seven days. Fortunately, it is rare, but it is very serious and requires urgent medical attention.

In any of the above circumstances, after first aid is administered, if indicated, the person should be taken to the nearest medical facility.[5]

Another possible complication resulting from alcohol abuse is that inebriated persons are often more inclined to injure themselves. As previously indicated, the suicide rate among alcoholics is extremely high. Thus, an officer should be aware of how to deal with a person who is threatening suicide. The following suggestions might be useful to remember when coming into contact with such a person.

1. Take all threats to commit suicide seriously.
2. Don't threaten someone who is threatening suicide.
3. Try to stimulate the "will to live" in the individual.
4. Don't make any sudden moves toward the person until you are close enough to grab hold of him.
5. Send someone to get professional assistance (clergyman, doctor) while you are speaking to him.[6]

Drinking and Driving

Drunkenness has long presented problems for drivers, those who don't mix drinking and driving as well as those who do. Drunken mothers were condemned by an eighteenth-century justice of the peace in England for allowing their children to dash about without supervision, thus leading to accidents resulting in broken carriages and injured horses. As most people realize, the situation has become drastically worse within the past few years. A recent report by the U.S. Department of Transportation estimates that alcohol is the precipitating factor in 800,000 automobile accidents and 28,000 automobile-related deaths each year, most of them occurring in the late afternoon or evening.

Though the National Safety Council has stated that alcoholics usually account for alcohol-related deaths on the highway, many accidents are still caused by nonalcoholics who drive under the influence of alcohol. Many drivers in this condition refuse to believe that as few as two drinks can cause impaired judgment, distorted vision, slower reaction time. They somehow feel that they are immune to the effects of alcohol; others may be influenced, but not them. However, when such drivers are stopped by the police and asked to take the drunk-driving test, they might be subject to harsh penalties if found to be inebriated.

At present, determining whether a person is too inebriated to drive is based on two legal decisions. One of these is a 1935 decision by the Arizona Supreme Court, which has been endorsed by the American Medical Association and the National Safety Council.

> The expression "under the influence of intoxicating liquor" covers not only all the well-known and easily recognizable conditions and degrees of intoxication, but also any abnormal mental or physical condition which is the result of indulging to any degree in intoxicating liquors and which tends to deprive the individual of that clearness of intellect and control of himself which he would otherwise possess. If the ability of the driver of an automobile has been lessened in the slightest degree by the use of intoxicating liquors, then the driver is deemed to be under the influence of intoxicating liquor. The mere fact that a driver has taken a drink does not place him under the ban of the statute unless such drink has some influence upon him, lessening in some degree his ability to handle said automobile.[7]

Most states have interpreted this decision in the following manner:

1. A blood-alcohol level of less than 0.05 percent means *no* intoxication.
2. A blood-alcohol level of between 0.05 and 0.15 percent indicates that the individual *may* be under the influence of alcohol.
3. A blood-alcohol level of over 0.15 percent is *prima facie* evidence that the person is intoxicated.

Detection and Primary Intervention. There are several instances in which a police officer is in a position to observe an intoxicated driver firsthand. These opportunities may arise when officers have positioned themselves in order to observe traffic flow, while on patrol, when in the process of stopping drivers for routine checks or when issuing citations for moving or nonmoving violations, and during an accident investigation.

While parked, officers can easily keep moving traffic under surveillance to spot hazardous or unusual operation of a vehicle. The signs the officers are looking for that would warrant stopping a motorist are fairly straightforward, for they are similar to the signs manifested by a driver under the influence of drugs, or by one who is an habitual reckless driver. (See Table 2.1.)

Once an officer has decided to stop a vehicle, he or she should signal the operator to pull over, and then watch for a number of possible reactions in addition to the normal one in which the driver pulls over correctly. These include failure to stop soon after being signaled; attempted escape; an abrupt stop in the middle of the road; and/or a swerving, dangerous stop. How the person reacts after being signaled to stop can provide the first clue that the person may be intoxicated. By the time the motorist has pulled off the road, the officer has already had time to gather information about the driver—based on the manner in which the driver was acting prior to being signaled to pull over and the way in which the driver responded once requested to stop.

The next set of clues can be observed just prior to the driver's exiting from the vehicle. First, the driver may attempt to change seats with the person in the passenger seat. The driver may also try to quickly conceal alcoholic beverages in the glove compartment, under the seat, or by throwing them out of the window; sometimes the motorist exits from the car immediately in an attempt

TABLE 2.1 SIGNS OF HAZARDOUS/UNUSUAL OPERATION OF A VEHICLE POSSIBLY INDICATING AN INTOXICATED DRIVER

Weaving in traffic	Cutting off other motorists
Ignoring traffic signals and signs	Skimming (touching slightly or almost hitting) parked cars
Driving too slowly	Driving without lights on
Speeding	Waiting a long period to start after light changes to green
Hazardous passing	Yelling obscene language or making obscene gestures
Running or overshooting stop signs	Failure to dim headlights when appropriate
Tailing	Driving with excessively dirty or blocked windows
Backing up without looking	Throwing objects from vehicle
Driving on wrong side of street	Drinking in the vehicle

to prove that everything is under control, and occasionally the driver may attempt to escape.

Once the officer comes into contact with the motorist, there are a number of signs that he or she should look for—again, these are usually quite evident and fairly easy to detect.

Some of the common physical signs of intoxication are:

1. Flushed, pale, or bruised face
2. Bloodshot or crossed eyes
3. Alcohol on the breath
4. Belching, hiccuping, vomiting, or shallow or heavy breathing
5. Uncoordinated gait, stumbling, walking into objects
6. Profuse sweating
7. Unkempt appearance
8. Incontinence
9. Uncontrollable waving of the arms and hands

Some of the common psychological signs of intoxication are:

1. Inappropriate laughing, crying, or talking
2. General hostility for no apparent reason
3. Incoherent speech or mumbling
4. General disorientation; the suspect may not know where he or she is or even the time of day
5. Inappropriate behavior in response to the officer's requests

If these signs are present they will be observable when the motorist gets out of the vehicle and responds to a request to show a driver's license and registration. (Naturally, officers should visually survey the inside of the vehicle and its other occupants when approaching the vehicle and during the initial contact with the motorist.) If the driver does not appear to be intoxicated (but possibly just sleepy from traveling for a long time), and if motor vehicle documents are in order and the driver hasn't broken any traffic laws, the driver would naturally be permitted to proceed—with a warning if it is deemed necessary.

If, on the other hand, the driver appears to be intoxicated, then the officer should immediately advise the driver of legal rights and ask the driver to move to an area away from the vehicle and moving traffic so that dexterity-physical coordination tests can be administered immediately. (See Table 2.2.)

If after these tests the officers feel that they do not have sufficient evidence of intoxication and if the driver appears sober enough to drive, but has broken a moving traffic law, a citation should be issued and the driver should be allowed to proceed. If enough evidence is present, the violator should be placed under arrest, handcuffed, searched for alcohol, drugs, and weapons, placed in the patrol car, and advised of legal rights under the so-called implied consent law. Following this procedure, any other occupants of the car should be interviewed, the suspect's car should be searched, and any evidence should be collected and receipted according to standard procedures. (See also sections in Chapter 10 which deal with collecting and preserving evidence.)

Following the arrest, the violator's car should be secured until it can be moved to safety. Arrangements must also be made for transportation of the other occupants of the car. The suspect should then be taken either to a

TABLE 2.2 EXAMPLES OF DEXTERITY/PHYSICAL COORDINATION TESTS ADMINISTERED TO SUSPECTED INTOXICATED DRIVERS

Romberg Test:	The suspect is asked to stand with feet together, arms at the side, and eyes closed, and to tilt the head ten seconds.
Finger-to-Nose Test:	Standing, feet together, eyes closed, and arms outstretched at a right angle to body, the suspect is asked to extend the index finger, making a fist with the rest of the fingers, and then to attempt to touch tip of the nose with the finger by bending the arm at elbow; this process is then repeated with the right arm.
Balancing on One Leg:	Standing, feet together, arms at the side, looking straight ahead, the suspect is asked to extend the left leg forward without bending it and to hold it approximately one foot off the ground for ten seconds; this process is then repeated with the right foot.
Walking a Straight Line:	The suspect is asked to walk heel to toe in a straight line for several steps, then to turn on command and walk heel to toe back to the original position.

hospital—in the event that there is a severe alcohol-related problem requiring immediate medical attention, such as alcohol hallucinosis or convulsions—or to a detention facility for chemical tests, temporary incarceration, if necessary, and the booking process.

During an accident investigation police officers must also suspect the possibility that one or more of the drivers involved might be under the influence of alcohol. In addition to the presence of open bottles in the vehicle, other signs which may indicate possible alcohol use on the part of a driver include failure to have lights on, reports by witnesses indicating that the driver was swerving or driving on the wrong side of the road, or an actual failure on the part of the motorist to comprehend how the accident occurred or that it even occurred at all (however, this sign may be a symptom of shock as well).

If officers are sensitive to the signs that a person is or has been drinking while driving, much can be done to prevent alcohol-related accidents. Of course, most states do have an efficient, well-organized training program for their officers in the area of detection, investigation, and arrest of intoxicated drivers. The job is mammoth, however, and the work of removing the intoxicated driver from the road is vitally important to driving safety. Therefore, the methods and techniques presented in this chapter are at the very least meant to reinforce this important police operation.

The other major decision affecting determination of inebriation is the implied consent law which was enacted in the state of New York in 1953.[8] This law contains two important provisions.

1. Upon receiving a permit to drive the motorist agrees as well to submit to a chemical test if so requested by an officer.
2. If the driver refuses to be tested for being under the influence of alcohol, his or her license can be revoked.

Finding New Solutions

License revocation, however, is certainly not the final answer to the problems caused by the drunken driver. Strict enforcement and publication of standardized penalties also play an important part. The driver must be discouraged from getting behind the wheel when intoxicated. Through public education, the drinker must be taught to leave the driving to one who is sober or avoid driving after having had too much to drink. Furthermore, repeated offenders must be taken off the road permanently before they cause that almost inevitable accident or death.

Public education of the hard-and-fast rules on mixing drinking and driving is one basic way of dealing with inebriated drivers. But dealing with the problems of handling the alcoholic or intoxicated person in the street is more complex. In theory, alcohol abusers should be diverted from the justice system, but instead they are funneled directly into it.

Possibly, at some point in time, alcohol abusers will be diverted to rehabilitation centers for outpatient care at an early stage. Using this approach, the first alcohol-related incident a person is involved in will be viewed not as a crime, but as a warning signal that treatment is needed. Until then, however, peace and police officers will be required to handle the bulk of the problem on a day-to-day basis. Accordingly, knowing something about the nature of alcohol and the complications which can arise from its abuse is not superfluous, but necessary.

Notes

1. National Institute of Mental Health, *Alcohol and Alcoholism* (Chevy Chase, Md.: NIMH, 1969), pp. 19–20.
2. Berton Roueche, *The Neutral Spirit: A Portrait of Alcohol* (Boston: Little, Brown, 1960), p. 17.
3. N. H. Clark, *The Dry Years: Prohibition and Social Change in Washington* (Seattle: University of Washington Press, 1965), p. 54.
4. President's Commission on Law Enforcement and Administration of Justice, *Task Force Report: Drunkenness* (Washington, D.C.: Government Printing Office, 1967), pp. 3–4.
5. The Correctional Association of New York and the International Association of Police Chiefs, *Alcohol and Alcoholism: A Police Handbook* (New York: Smithers Foundation, 1965), pp. 24–26.
6. Robert J. Wicks, *Applied Psychology for Law Enforcement and Correction Officers* (New York: McGraw-Hill, 1974), p. 87.
7. *Steffani v. State,* 40 orig. 210. 42P. 2d 615 (1936), p. 618.
8. New York Vehicle and Traffic Law of 1929, Section 7(a), as added by L. 1953, c. 854.

Selected Bibliography

American Medical Association. *Chemical Tests for Intoxication*. Chicago: A.M.A., 1959.

______. *Manual on Alcoholism*. Chicago: A.M.A., 1967.

______. *Alcohol and the Impaired Driver*. Chicago: A.M.A., 1968.

______. *Breath/Alcohol Tests*. Chicago: A.M.A., 1972.

Correctional Association of New York and the International Association of Police Chiefs. *Alcohol and Alcoholism: A Police Handbook*. New York: Smithers Foundation, 1965.

Fox, B., and Rox, J. H., eds. *Alcohol and Traffic Safety*. Bethesda, Md.: U.S. Department of Health, Education, and Welfare, 1963.

Fox, R., ed. *Alcoholism*. New York: Springer, 1967.

Julien, R. M. *A Primer of Drug Action*. San Francisco: Freeman, 1975.

Leavitt, F. *Drugs and Behavior*. Philadelphia: Saunders, 1974.

National Highway Traffic Safety Administration and Michigan State University Highway Traffic Safety Center. *DWI Law Enforcement Training Project Student Manual*. Washington, D.C.: U.S. Government Printing Office, 1974.

Ray, O. S. "Alcohol," in *Drugs, Society, and Human Behavior*. St. Louis: Mosby, 1972.

Wicks, R. J. "Alcoholism," In *Applied Psychology for Law Enforcement and Correction Officers*. New York: McGraw-Hill, 1974.

Chapter 3

Depressants: Barbiturates, Tranquilizers, and Inhalants

Alcohol, as indicated in Chapter 2, is perhaps the most widely abused depressant in this country. But alcohol is only one of the many depressant substances which are subject to widespread abuse. A more complete list should include the following:

1. Alcohol
2. Barbiturates
   a. Amobarbital (trade name: Amytal)
   b. Pentobarbital (trade name: Nembutal)
   c. Phenobarbital (trade name: Luminal)
   d. Secobarbital (trade name: Seconal)
3. Nonbarbiturate Depressants.
   a. Chloral hydrate
   b. Paraldehyde
   c. Ethchlorvynol (trade name: Placidyl)
   d. Ethinamate (trade name: Valmid)
   e. Glutethimide (trade name: Doriden)
   f. Methaqualone (trade names: Quaalude, Somnafac, Sopor)
   g. Methyprylon (trade name: Noludar)
4. Tranquilizers
   a. Meprobamate (trade names: Miltown, Equanil)
   b. Chlordiazepoxide (trade name: Librium)
   c. Diazepam (trade name: Valium)

The solvents and inhalants also belong in this category, but because of their nature and mode of use they will be discussed in a separate section of this chapter.

Behavioral Depressants

Barbiturates, nonbarbiturate hypnotics (sedatives), and tranquilizers all have one characteristic in common—they reduce one's levels of alertness and activity. For this reason they are referred to collectively as the *behavioral depressants*. The effects of these drugs vary in degree depending upon the *amount* of the substance taken as well as its *potency* or strength.

Small amounts of the more potent substances, such as the barbiturates, or larger amounts of the less potent substances, such as the tranquilizers, generally bring relief from emotional upset or anxiety. This effect is known as *tranquilization*—hence, the term "tranquilizers." With larger doses, *sedation* or an even greater depression of the level of emotional reactivity and alertness to the environment occurs. Finally, with sufficiently large doses, sleep is induced. Drugs that induce sleep are called *hypnotics*. When taken in even larger doses than those required to induce sleep, they prevent the user from feeling physical pain, and thus act as *anesthetics*. According to one text on drug action,

> depending upon the dose, any sedative-hypnotic compound may be classified as a sedative, a tranquilizer, a hypnotic, or an anesthetic. The compounds differ, therefore, from one another, not in their sites of actions, uses, or abilities to induce various stages of depression, but in their individual potency and in the chemical differences that cause them to be handled differently by the body.[1]

The stages of intoxication experienced by a person using any of the depressant drugs are not dissimilar from those described for alcohol in Chapter 2. At low doses all of these substances, although in fact depressants, are capable of producing varying degrees of excitement, euphoria, and loss of inhibitions. As in the case of alcohol, what is actually happening is that the inhibitory or control centers of the brain are themselves being inhibited by the depressant action of these substances. Freed from their restraining action, there is less control over the excitatory processes in the brain, which in turn produces a sense of euphoria in the user. With even greater doses of the drug, however, the action of these excitatory elements becomes inhibited and sleep eventually results.

Because the modes of action of the various drugs discussed in this chapter are so similar, certain common characteristics—in addition to those already mentioned—can be delineated for all of them. These characteristics include the following:

1. *Potential for Addiction*. All of the sedatives described here are potentially highly addicting. Their repeated use in large doses may lead to increasing *tolerance* and possibly the development of *physical dependency*—the user requires larger and larger doses in order to obtain the desired effects and physical illness may occur upon discontinuance. Barbiturate addiction may even be compared to opiate addiction in that a single dose may lead to the development of some tolerance.[2] As in the case of opiate addiction, discontinuation of use may result in the appearance of the *abstinence syndrome,* in this case called the *general depressant withdrawal syndrome*. This syndrome is characterized by nervousness, anxiety, weakness, and inability to sleep. Individuals who use barbiturates

daily in doses of six-tenths of a gram over a period of one to two months have about a 50 percent chance of experiencing these symptoms upon discontinuation of the drug. In more severe cases of addiction, seizures and convulsions may be present.

In addition to the development of physical dependence, a strong *psychological dependence* may be present, particularly in individuals who regularly use sedatives to induce sleep.

There may also be a tendency among persons who frequently use depressants (such as barbiturates) to induce sleep to begin using stimulants in order to neutralize the hangover effects of the sedative. This not uncommon practice leads to the development of a pattern of cyclical drug abuse.

There is also evidence that the quality of sleep obtained with barbiturates is different from that of normal, nonbarbiturate sleep. During typical barbiturate sleep, there is a significant decrease in the amount of dreaming that takes place. When barbiturate use ceases, this dreaming time is "made up" and sleep may be disturbed by intense dreams.

2. *Interchangeability of Depressants.* Because all the depressants act in similar ways, the state of intoxication produced by one is much like that produced by another. Accordingly, these drugs may be used interchangeably to prevent withdrawal symptoms. (It should be noted, however, that barbiturates are not effective in staving off withdrawal from heroin, indicating that these two classes of drugs probably act upon different parts of the brain.

   Some persons may combine the use of two or more of these drugs—for example, alcohol and barbiturates. Barbiturates may also be used along with heroin to produce a more intense "high." In such use, the effects of the two drugs are *additive,* the effect of both being greater than either one by itself.

3. *Antagonistic Action toward Stimulants.* The effects of the depressants are antagonistic to those of the stimulants. That is, each of these classes of drugs neutralizes the effects of the other. Thus, the depressants may be used to bring one down from the high produced by one of the amphetamines ("uppers"), or by cocaine. (Hence, the depressants are known as "downers.") Unfortunately, however, this practice is not as effective when attempting to revive a person from a depressed state—in fact, administering a stimulant to such a person might result in an even deeper depression. Of course, downers are also used to remove one from a normal state of arousal, and some persons use them specifically for this purpose, particularly those who ingest large doses of depressant drugs.

Abuse of Barbiturates and Tranquilizers

The pattern of abuse observed in barbiturate and tranquilizer users is quite different from that observed in heroin and cocaine users, at least in the early stages. It more closely resembles the pattern seen in the nonheroin opiate addict who becomes addicted while using morphine or some other opiate for the relief of pain. Most barbiturate abusers are older than heroin users and are likely to have begun using barbiturates for medical reasons—for instance, to induce sleep. Likewise, the use of tranquilizers often begins as a means of controlling anxiety. While using these drugs, an individual may discover that they not only relieve the initial complaint, but also induce a pleasant state of intoxication, which may eventually become the desired effect. Thereupon, the intake of the drug is increased until it levels off, and the user will seek out a continued supply, either through legitimate channels or from "pushers." Finding a source for the drug will assume an urgency similar to that observed in the opiate addict who suddenly finds—perhaps the first time he or she runs out of the drug—that it is very difficult to live without it. At this point, the tranquilizer user is "hooked."

Of course, there are sedative addicts who use the drug only on weekends or for longer periods of time intermittently. Others may use only a small amount of the drug, adjusting their dosage to the level of euphoria they desire.

Side Effects and Medical Complications

The long-term outcome of using depressant drugs regularly is similar to that of long-term alcohol use described in Chapter 2. Malnutrition may occur; social functioning may be totally disrupted—the addict will not be able to work or maintain a normal family life; seizures resembling delirium tremens may occur during withdrawal.

On a more immediate basis, abuse of the depressant drugs again presents a similar picture to that seen with alcohol. Driving ability is impaired during intoxication, and hangovers may occur. There is also a much greater risk of accidental death from overdose with use of these drugs because their potency is greater and because extremely large doses may be inadvertently taken when they are in the form of capsules. The depressants are also commonly used in deliberate suicide attempts.

Minor Tranquilizers

During the past twenty years, a class of drugs known as the minor tranquilizers has come into wide use. This class of drugs, which includes such widely known substances as meprobamate (Miltown, Equanil), chlordiazepoxide (Librium), and diazepam (Valium), is used to alleviate the symptoms of anxiety and tension. The earliest of the three to be used, meprobamate, was originally introduced as a muscle relaxant, but in fact it did not act as a muscle relaxant. Neither is it actually a tranquilizer in the true sense of the term. Rather, its characteristics, as well as those of chlordiazepoxide and diazepam, are very similar to those of the barbiturates. At low doses, they induce relief from anxiety and tension, and a sense of well-being; at high doses, they induce sleep. The minor tranquilizers do tend to work for a long period of time—sometimes up to ten or twelve hours.

The pattern of abuse associated with the minor tranquilizers is almost identical to that described for the barbiturates. Similarly, all that was said earlier regarding tolerance, dependency (physiological and psychological), and withdrawal also applies. A major difference between barbiturates and minor tranquilizers is that the more potent barbiturates present a greater risk of overdose.

Methods of Administration

The barbiturates and minor tranquilizers are almost always taken orally, because they are usually available in capsule or tablet form. Occasionally, one may hear of them being injected subcutaneously, and this mode of administration is more likely to be associated with the barbiturates. In contrast to the minor tranquilizers, which all tend to be long-acting, the barbiturates vary markedly in their length of action. Phenobarbital (Luminal) is a long-acting barbiturate while amobarbital (Amytal), an intermediate barbiturate, has a shorter duration of action, and pentobarbital (Nembutal) and secobarbital (Seconal) act for an even shorter period of time. The effects of a long-acting barbiturate may last up to ten hours; an intermediate-acting one to five hours; and a short-acting one to two or three hours.

Nonbarbiturate Depressants

The nonbarbiturate depressants include such substances as chloral hydrate, paraldehyde, the bromides, glutethimide (Doriden), and methaqualone. The first three of these substances were used for many years as "sleeping potions." Of the three, chloral hydrate is probably the most well known because when added to alcohol it induces sleep. This is known as the "Mickey Finn" cocktail. However, because of the unpleasant taste of chloral hydrate and paraldehyde, and some unpleasant side effects of the former, they are rarely used today. The bromides also have unpleasant side effects. Glutethimide (Doriden) is another depressant drug that is used to induce sleep. It has been advertised as being a nonbarbiturate, but in reality it has a similar chemical structure and produces similar effects.

Of all of the nonbarbiturate sedatives, methaqualone (Quaalude, Sopor, Somnafac) is the one that is commonly abused—most especially by young people. Developed some twenty-five years ago, it has recently become a particularly favored sedative of abuse. Often taken orally in social settings, the state of intoxication resulting from ingestion of the drug is called "luding out," particularly when it is taken with wine. The drug is believed to enhance sexual performance, but in reality it merely lowers inhibitions while at the same time decreasing capacity. Both tolerance and physical dependence have been reported in methaqualone use, and it is considered to have high abuse and addiction potential.

Inhalants

Inhalants are substances whose vapors, when inhaled, produce a change in the conscious state of the mind. They include:

1. Toluene (plastic cement and paint thinner)
2. Gasoline
3. Trichloroethylene (cleaning fluid, spot remover)
4. Acetone (paint remover, nail polish remover)
5. Naphtha (cigarette and charcoal lighter fluids and some glues; paint removers)
6. Fluorocarbons (aerosol propellants)

The deliberate use of such products as model airplane glue, plastic cement, lighter fluid, gasoline, and related substances to obtain a high represents a relatively new area of drug abuse. However, inhaling certain chemicals for specific effects dates back some years. Nitrous oxide (laughing gas) was being used to produce intoxication as early as the 1800s. Today's abuse of inhalants differs in several significant ways from the patterns of abuse associated with other substances we have discussed so far. First, the primary abusers of these substances are generally younger than abusers of other drugs, most of them being in their early teens or even preteens. Second, most of the substances being abused are readily available, having few if any legal restrictions upon their distribution—in the few instances in which restrictions do exist, they can be easily circumvented. Finally, some of these substances have an extremely high potential for causing illness or even death.

How Inhalants Produce Intoxication

The vapors of all the products mentioned above (it should be noted that this list is far from comprehensive) are central nervous system depressants, and act in much the same way as do alcohol and the barbiturates. They produce a state of euphoria by initially depressing inhibiting centers in the central nervous system, thus producing a general euphoria. However, other effects are likely to result from use of inhalants. One medical textbook lists the following symptoms as occurring upon inhaling gasoline: "incoordination, restlessness, excitement, confusion, disorientation, ataxia, delirium, and finally, coma that may last for a few hours to several days."[4] Another source describes the additional effects as "ranging from a simple somnolence and dizziness to delusions of unusual strength or the ability to fly to outright visual and auditory hallucinations similar to those experienced with the ingestion of psychotomimetic agents."[5]

The effects produced by inhaling, or "sniffing," these substances are relatively short-lived, usually lasting less than an hour and then wearing off after a period of drowsiness, which may last up to several hours. However, there may be certain side effects, including vomiting, diarrhea, nausea, and chest pains.

Other symptoms, similar to those seen in the common cold—coughing, sneezing, tearing of the eyes, and runny nose—may also be present. Most of these side effects soon disappear.

Are Inhalants Addicting?

It is known that tolerance can occur with continued use of most of the substances used as inhalants. The development of physical dependence, however, has not been reported, and there is no reason to believe it exists. Psychological dependence, on the other hand, may occur.

The Dangers of Inhalants

Some volatile substances such as naphtha, petroleum distillates, and toluene are less toxic than others—for example, trichloroethylene (used in cleaning fluids) and the fluorinated hydrocarbons (used as aerosol propellants or refrigerants), both of which may cause disturbances of heart functioning. Other substances, such as carbon tetrachloride (used as a cleaning fluid or spot remover), the glycols contained in antifreeze, and some other substances used in plastic cements—for example, methyl cellosolve acetate—are potential causes for serious damage to the internal organs, including the kidneys, liver, brain, and other organs. Disorders of the blood may also result. One disorder associated with gasoline intoxication appears to be lead poisoning.

In addition to the direct toxic effects of the substances themselves, of which trichloroethane and fluorohydrocarbon seem to produce the most adverse effects, many of the dangers associated with these compounds are indirect. For instance, while intoxicated, youngsters may be injured during activities such as bike riding which under normal circumstances would not be considered dangerous. They might also be burned when volatile substances ignite. Finally, they might inadvertently suffocate while inhaling glue or some other substance from a bag.

Notes

1. R. M. Julien, *A Primer of Drug Action* (San Francisco: Freeman, 1975), p. 42.
2. S. K. Sharpless, "Hypnotics and Sedatives: Part I. The Barbiturates," in L. S. Goodman and A. Gilman, eds., *Pharmacological Basis of Therapeutics,* 4th ed. (New York: Macmillan, 1970), p. 108.
3. Jaffe, J. H. "Drug Addiction and Drug Abuse," in Goodman and Gilman, *Pharmacological Basis of Therapeutics,* p. 290.
4. E. A. Swinyard, "Noxious Gases and Vapors," in Goodman and Gilman, *Pharmacological Basis of Therapeutics,* p. 937.
5. F. G. Hofmann, *A Handbook on Drug and Alcohol Abuse: The Biomedical Aspects* (New York: Oxford, 1975), p. 135.

Selected Bibliography

Angrist, B., Rotrosen, J., and Gershon, S. "Assessment of Tolerance to the Hallucinogenic Effects of DOM." *Psychopharmacology* 36 (1974): 203–207.

Assig, C. "Drug Dependence of the Barbiturate Type." *Drug Dependence* 5 (1970): 24–27.

Cappell, H.; LeBlanc, A. E.; and Endrenyi, L. "Aversive Conditioning by Psychoactive Drugs: Effects of Morphine, Alcohol, and Chlordiazepoxide." *Psychopharmacology* (1973): 239–246.

DiGiacomo, J. N., and King, C. L. "Codeine and Glutethimide Addiction." *International Journal of the Addictions* 5 (1970): 279–285.

Gray, G. R.; Smith, D. E.; Wesson, D.; and Sheppard, C. "A New Method of Outpatient Treatment of Barbiturate Withdrawal." *Journal of Psychedelic Drugs* 3 (1971): 81–88.

Gray, G. R.; Smith, D. E.; Wesson, D. R.; and Sheppard, C. W. "Outpatient Barbiturate Withdrawal Using Phenobarbital," *International Journal of the Addictions* 7 (1972): 17–26.

Hartmann, E., and Cravens, J. "The Effects of Long-term Administration of Psychotropic Drugs on Human Sleep. V. The Effects of Chloral Hydrate." *Psychopharmacology* 33 (1973): 219–232.

Hartmann, E., and Cravens, J. "The Effects of Long-term Administration of Psychotropic Drugs on Human Sleep. VI. The Effects of Chlordiazepoxide," *Psychopharmacology* 33 (1973): 233–245.

Inaba, D. S.; Ray, G. R.; Newmeyer, J. A.; and Whitehead, C. "Methaqualone Abuse. 'Luding Out.'," *Journal of the American Medical Association* 224 (1973): 1505–1509.

Kunnes, R. "Methaqualone Addiction: Institutional Non-Response." *Contemporary Drug Problems* 2 (1973): 47–50.

Linnoila, M., and Häkkinen, S. "Effects of Diazepam and Codeine, Alone and in Combination with Alcohol, on Simulated Driving." *Clinical Pharmacology and Therapeutics* 15 (1974): 368–373.

Mehar, G. S.; Parker, J. M.; and Tubas, T. "Interaction Between Alcohol, Minor Tranquilizers and Morphine," *International Journal of Clinical Pharmacology, Therapeutics and Toxicology* 9 (1974): 70–74.

Pascarelli, E. F. "Methaqualone Abuse, the Quiet Epidemic," *Journal of the American Medical Association* 224 (1973): 1512–1514.

Spear, P. W., and Protass, L. M. "Barbiturate Poisoning—An Endemic Disease. Five Years Experience in a Municipal Hospital." *Medical Clinics of North America* 57 (1973): 1471–1479.

Tennant, F. S. "Complications of Methaqualone-Diphenhydramine (Mandrax) Abuse." *British Journal of Addiction* 69 (1973): 327–330.

Chapter 4
Opiates

If the vast array of commonly abused drugs could be metaphorically likened to the members of a kingdom, then surely their monarch would be ''King Heroin.'' In recent years, heroin has probably received more attention from hard-drug users, investigators, and treatment agencies than has any other drug currently available.

During the past decade, the psychophysiological actions of heroin have been carefully studied, its users' personalities and responses to treatment have been scrutinized, and an array of legal measures have been enacted in an effort to curb its use.

Even poetry has been written about it.

King Heroin

Beware my friend
My name is King Heroin.
Where I come from everybody knows.
I come from the land where the poppy seeds grow.

I entered this country without a passport.
Ever since then I've been hunted and sought,
By junkies, addicts and plainclothes dicks,
But mostly by a sick junkie who needs a quick fix.

My little white grains are nothing but waste.
I'm soft and bitter and deadly to taste.
I'm worlds powerful, all know it's true.
Use me just once and you'll know it's true.

I'll make a schoolboy forget about his books.
And I'll cause a world beauty to neglect her looks.
I'll make a good husband cast away his wife,
And send a greedy pusher away for life.

I'm king of crime, prince of corruption.
I'll capture your soul and cause your destruction.
More precious than diamonds, more treasured than gold,
My value to some is brutally told.

Ahhh! The police have taken you from under my wing.
They dare defy me, I who am King.
They have taken you from me for a short rest,
But they cannot rule me, for I am the best.

You'll curse my name and down me in speech,
But you would pick me up again if I were in reach.
At night while you're sleeping and planning your fate,
You know I'll be waiting just beyond the gate.

I gave you warning, but you didn't heed.
So put your foot in my stirrup and ride my steed.
When you ride me you'll ride me well
On the White Horse of Heroin, you'll ride me to Hell.

Anonymous

Reading the poem "King Heroin" can give one a sense of the insidious power of heroin; one can begin to understand the potential impact of this dangerous narcotic on the person who uses it. However, to gain a more comprehensive understanding of exactly what heroin is, how and whom it affects, and why, a knowledge of the facts and various theories advanced by researchers is also needed. Therefore, the first part of this chapter will provide information on how heroin is manufactured, how it produces its effects, and the methods by which it is used.

What Is Heroin?

Heroin is a narcotic. In its pure form it is a white, bitter, odorless crystalline compound known to chemists as *diacetylmorphine*. But this form is rarely seen—either by the Asian, Middle Eastern and Mexican growers of the opium poppy from which the drug is derived or by users on the street. In order for the substance to reach a pure crystalline powder form, it must pass through a number of stages.

1. The poppy plant (*Papaver somniferum*) produces a milky substance.
2. This substance is dried and made into a powder (opium).
3. Morphine is extracted from the opium.
4. Morphine through exposure to acetic acid produces heroin.

Heroin in its pure form rarely if ever reaches the street user. Rather, it is cut (diluted or mixed) with such noxious substances as quinine and lactose, or a dangerous substance such as rat poison. By cutting the heroin with harmless mixtures, the drug pusher can increase the quantity of "street heroin" and raise the ultimate return on the original investment. On the other hand, by mixing the heroin with a harmful agent such as rat poison or by selling a dose of unusually high purity, the pusher can eliminate an undesirable user.

The strength or purity of street heroin is questionable; the user is never really sure how potent it is. But, in most cases, the one thing that the addict can be sure of is that the heroin being sold today is not as strong as the heroin that was available in the past. Unlike the 1920s and 1930s when it was possible to obtain heroin that was 60 to 80 percent pure, the street heroin that is available today is usually less than 2 percent pure. Because most street heroin is so greatly adulterated with other substances, "shooting-up" with unusually pure heroin may result in death from an overdose.

How Heroin Is Used

Heroin can be taken orally ("dropped"), sniffed ("snorted"), smoked, or injected—either under the skin ("skin-popping") or directly into the veins ("mainlining"). Currently, the most popular method of taking the drug is mainlining. The preference for mainlining is not surprising, considering the scarcity of pure heroin in the street form and the fact that injecting the drug intravenously produces a more pronounced initial effect than do the other methods of use. However, among American soldiers in Southeast Asia, where pure heroin was readily available, smoking was the preferred method of use.

The drug is prepared for injection by heating a solution of street heroin and water in a "cooker"—that is, a spoon or bottlecap. This mixture is then drawn up through a needle into a syringe or eyedropper. (Often a cotton pledget is put into the mixture; this serves as a filter.) A tourniquet, belt, heavy rubber band, or similar device is then wrapped around the arm or leg to raise the veins so that the solution can be injected into the body.

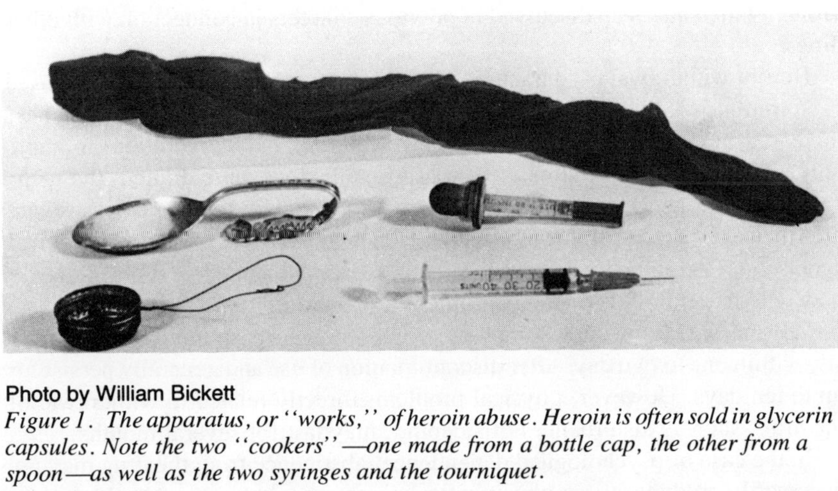

Photo by William Bickett

Figure 1. The apparatus, or "works," of heroin abuse. Heroin is often sold in glycerin capsules. Note the two "cookers"—one made from a bottle cap, the other from a spoon—as well as the two syringes and the tourniquet.

Addiction: Tolerance and Dependence

Heroin, as an opiate and central nervous system depressant, can produce a number of physical effects. The degree and duration of these effects depends on a number of factors, including method of administration, size and purity of the dose, and the amount of prior experience the user has had with opiates. Research has shown that heroin moves to the brain more rapidly than does morphine; however, once there, it is broken down into an intermediate product and then into morphine; it is this latter substance that accounts for most of the effects the user experiences. One of the differences between heroin and morphine is that heroin produces a much more rapid onset of action or ''jolt'' (also known as a ''rush''). This is the result of heroin's comparatively rapid entry from the bloodstream into the brain.

Among the effects of heroin are pain reduction, euphoria, relief from diarrhea, constipation, drowsiness, pupil constriction, and a decrease in the rate of respiration. (The decreased rate of respiration is a sign that anyone having contact with drug users should be particularly aware of, because an overdose can produce respiratory arrest, stoppage of breathing, and even death.)

Two other results of continued heroin use are the development of physiological tolerance and psychophysiological dependence. Persons who use heroin on a regular basis find it necessary to gradually increase their dose in order to achieve the desired effects; when this occurs, drug tolerance is said to be present.

As stated already, drug dependence can be both physiological and psychological in nature. In the case of heroin use, both types of dependence are present. Physical dependence on a drug is said to exist when a number of symptoms develop upon discontinuation of the drug. In the case of heroin, these symptoms constitute what is referred to as the withdrawal or abstinence syndrome, which has been discussed in previous chapters in connection with other drugs.

Heroin withdrawal is characterized by such symptoms as nausea, increased perspiration, ''goose flesh,'' anxiety, crying spells, irritability, body aches, increased blood pressure and heart rate, insomnia, and dehydration, to name only a few. Because the street heroin now available is quite diluted, the withdrawal or abstinence syndrome commonly seen today is somewhat less severe than that seen in the past. Moreover, with the increasing use of pharmacological agents such as methadone and nalorphine, treatment centers and hospitals are now able to detoxify the drug user much less painfully than in the past.

The major recognizable symptoms of withdrawal reach their highest intensity within one to two days after discontinuation of use and generally persist for up to ten days. However, physical problems directly related to withdrawal of the drug, such as disturbances of sleeping, may last for several months.

In the case of psychological dependence, abstinence from the drug may not necessarily produce strong physiological symptoms, but will cause the person to feel considerable emotional discomfort. Persons who are psychologically dependent on the drug may see its use as a means of achieving a more trouble-free life; because of this strong need for the pleasurable effects of the drug (at least during the early stages of its use), the time involved in obtaining and using it, and the personal inadequacies it circumvents, the user may feel compelled to continue its use—often such users convince themselves that they can stop using the drug whenever they want to.

Since *addiction* is considered by most researchers to be present when *a person develops tolerance to a drug and shows withdrawal symptoms and a pronounced desire to take it again after it has been discontinued for a period of time,* one can easily see how heroin qualifies as an addicting drug. Furthermore, because of heroin's unusually strong addiction potential, it requires special types of treatment and legal curbs and controls.

Side Effects and Medical Complications

The use of street heroin is a highly risky practice because it carries with it a substantial likelihood of causing disease, physical illness, and even death. The risk of contracting disease or developing an illness, however, is not a direct result of the effects of heroin itself, but is more often related to other factors—for example, the dangerous additives contained in street heroin, the unsanitary methods used to administer the drug, and the disregard by the addict for personal hygiene and nutrition. In addition to these factors, the addict of course can never determine the purity of the heroin contained in the "bag" just purchased, and therefore he or she runs the risk of overdosing.

In general, addicts have a higher death rate and a shorter life expectancy than nonaddicts. In fact, it has been estimated that as many as ten out of every 1,000 addicts die each year. One study indicated that the average life expectancy of male addicts entering the U.S. Public Health Service Hospital at Lexington, Kentucky, had already decreased by one-third by the time of their first admission. The life expectancy of female addicts had decreased by one-fifth.[1]

Addicts tend to die of a greater variety of illnesses than do nonaddicts.[2] They are more prone to infectious diseases such as tuberculosis and other lung diseases (including pneumonia), infections of the heart and kidneys, hepatitis, and tetanus. All of these diseases can be attributed to the use of heroin, which significantly lowers the addict's resistance to infection. One of the most common physical complications resulting from heroin addiction is the characteristic "railroad tracks," caused by repeated puncturing of the veins. These scars may be found anywhere on the body. More frequently found, however, are abscesses resulting from infections caused by bacteria present on contaminated needles. These are most often found in skin-poppers. Tattoos are sometimes used by addicts to camouflage the scars caused by repeated injections.

Overdosing, which frequently occurs in addicts, may be the result of one or more of the following:

1. Lack of knowledge of the content of the "bag."
2. Resuming use of high doses of the drug after a period of abstinence during which tolerance has been lowered—for example, following incarceration or detoxification.
3. The use of high doses of the drug by inexperienced persons.
4. The deliberate attempt by a dealer to eliminate an addict.
5. The purchase by an unwitting user of an unusually pure dose.

Death as a result of overdosing is generally caused by a depression of the vital breathing centers located in the brain stem.

Finally, addicts are more prone to death by other causes, such as suicide, accidents, and murder, than are nonaddicts. All in all, heroin addiction involves a high degree of risk.

Theories of Addiction

Given the many dangers and highly addicting properties of heroin, one naturally wonders why people use and continue to use it. The popular view is that heroin use is linked to one or more of the following:

1. The euphoric qualities of the drug.
2. Ignorance of the effects of long-term use.
3. The relief of pain, anxiety, or depression.
4. The fact that it allows the user to escape from the demands of the real world.
5. Becoming part of the in-group.
6. As a step up from other drugs.
7. Peer-group pressure.

Researchers have developed a number of theories to explain the widespread use of heroin. These theories can be broken down into three general categories: physiological, psychological, and sociological. Although no one theory supplies all the answers, these theories provide a framework for approaching the question of why people use heroin, and thus should be viewed in this light.

Recent physiological theories contend that narcotic addiction is closely tied to an unspecified metabolic deficiency. According to this view, a person may initially try heroin simply out of a desire to experiment with drugs, but it is a "neurological susceptibility" of some sort that accounts for the subsequent development of addiction.

The most widely accepted psychological theories of addiction are the psychoanalytic theory and the social-learning theory. As one might expect, the psychoanalytic theory is quite complex and relies on an understanding and acceptance of basic analytic principles. Since it cannot be easily applied to an appreciation of the problem of addiction or to the treatment of addicts, it is currently receiving little attention.

In the case of the social-learning theory of drug addiction, the models used are based on principles of conditioning. Although the theory is also too involved for an in-depth explanation here, it basically views drugs as being either directly or indirectly reinforcing. For example, persons who take drugs may be reinforced (or rewarded) for their behavior by experiencing a relief from pain or by gaining the acceptance of their peers.

The sociological theories of addiction are as numerous and complex as those belonging to the other two categories. But perhaps the most widely accepted sociological theory is the one advanced by A. R. Lindesmith, which can be summarized as follows:

1. *Initial Drug Use.* The person takes available drugs, often in response to pressure from peers, for any of a number of reasons (for example, pleasure); the user at this stage does not consider himself or herself an addict.
2. *Continued Drug Use.* The person is prompted to continue "getting high," unless the cost of buying drugs is so prohibitive as to produce a negative reaction, thus preventing further drug-taking behavior.
3. *"Hooked."* The user begins to experience withdrawal symptoms when his or her intake of narcotics is reduced or discontinued.
4. *Advanced Drug Behavior.* The addict now sees drugs as a solution to all problems—not only those caused by the distress of withdrawal, but those caused by stress in general. Increased dosage is prompted not only by a physiological need, but also by an increased sensitivity to the signs of imminent withdrawal.
5. *Revolving Door.* The user attempts to "cure" himself or herself in order to avoid the stigma of being labeled an "addict." But the stress of withdrawal, the isolation from society, and the loss of opportunities for advancement (occupational and/or social) may lead to an increased sense of failure and the eventual acceptance of oneself as an addict.[3]

A number of other sociologically oriented theories, which have gained widespread acceptance in recent years, are those that view drug abuse as a form of *deviant* behavior. These theories are primarily concerned with identifying and understanding the various factors that lead a person to engage in socially unacceptable behavior—in this case, excessive drug-taking. Why, they ask, do some people abuse drugs whereas others follow more conventional social norms? Several major factors have been identified to explain what causes a person to engage in drug-taking behavior.

1. Normal success channels are blocked or difficult to follow, thus leading the individual to seek out other means of self-fulfillment.
2. Membership in a valued peer group is easily accomplished by taking drugs; for such an individual, membership in accepted societal groups is usually either inaccessible or only remotely possible.
3. Acceptable goals are not easily achieved by legitimate means because of socioeconomic or personality barriers.

4. The individual is not punished for drug-taking behavior, and thus the negative outcome in the individual's behavior is not always apparent.
5. Little or no value is placed on conventional social norms, and membership in major societal groups may even be seen as undesirable.
6. Urban anonymity creates less need for conformity.
7. The easy availability of drugs to provide satisfaction, coupled with a lack of opportunity to find pleasure and fulfillment through legitimate channels, prompts the individual to follow the most accessible course of action—that is, taking drugs.

While all the theories described above can offer valuable insights into the nature of the problem of drug addiction, none of them offers a complete answer. Perhaps the main reason for the failure of any one theory to attract wide support and recognition is the fact that the addict population is itself not homogeneous. For example, although many addicts exhibit pathological traits and tend to become involved in criminal activities, this is not the case for all addicts; moreover, those who do exhibit psychopathological characteristics do not necessarily share the same ones. Thus, to accept the existence of an "addictive personality" or to see all addicts as potential criminals would be an error of oversimplification. Accordingly, it would be very difficult to devise a comprehensive theory to account for all aspects of the problem of addiction.

Characteristics of Heroin Users

Although it is extremely difficult to generalize about the types of individuals who become heroin addicts, it is nevertheless possible to identify a number of characteristics which seem to be shared by a large percentage of these individuals.

Family Environment. The family environments in which addicts spend their early childhood are frequently, but not always, characterized by poor parental adjustment and overall instability—for example, separated or divorced parents, emotionally distant or hostile fathers, and frequent illnesses or deaths among parents, especially among fathers.

Among the brothers and sisters of addicts, many are likely to have been arrested, or to have used drugs, perhaps in as many as four out of ten cases. Two out of ten are likely to have used heroin.[4]

Age. Addicts tend to be young adults, and the current trend seems to indicate that the average age is becoming lower. One recent study showed that whereas the average age of addicts in 1960 was twenty-eight, by 1973 the average had fallen to twenty-one.[5]

The age of nineteen has been suggested by one writer as the age of greatest susceptibility to heroin use.[6] In another study with similar findings, about two-thirds of male addicts had started using heroin before the age of twenty-one.[7] One of the authors has interviewed several addicts who began using heroin before the age of thirteen.

There are few older addicts. Most addicts use heroin for less than ten years, and only 8 percent of addicts are over thirty years of age.[8]

Sex. Most heroin addicts are male. Estimates of the percentage of female addicts usually are less than 20 percent.

Marital Status. Most addicts are unmarried, and when they are married the quality of their marriages is often poor.

Socioeconomic Status. A high proportion of addicts come from the most socioeconomically deprived segments of our society, although all social-class levels are represented. Minority groups tend to be overrepresented among addicts, probably as a result of the large minority-group population in urban poverty areas, and the frequently greater alienation from society felt by members of these groups.

Education. Although many studies have shown addicts to have poorer educational backgrounds than nonaddicts, no less than four recent studies have found this *not* to be the case.*

Intelligence. Here again, there are many conflicting reports. Some studies have shown addicts to have lower intelligence levels than nonaddicts, whereas others have shown that there are no differences in intelligence between the two groups.*

The problems of developing a theory become even more evident when one tries to describe narcotic addicts as a group. Descriptive analysis of a group is much easier than theoretical analysis. Yet, when one tries to describe addicts as a group of individuals who come from broken homes, who have lower I.Q.s, or who often have a previous history of criminality, one sometimes runs into research findings that contradict these claims. As a result, one can only view current theories of addiction as tentative stepping stones for future ideas, since to accept them with any greater degree of certitude would be a mistake.

Heroin Use and Criminality

Are all addicts criminals? Does heroin use lead to criminal behavior? These questions are frequently asked by personnel in criminal justice and correctional fields. Naturally, the answers to these questions are extremely relevant to effective law enforcement.

With respect to the first question, the fact is that most heroin users, though not all, have a history of criminal behavior. In fact, some studies have shown

*See Platt and Labate's *Heroin Addiction* for a more detailed discussion of these issues.

that as many as 80 to 90 percent of addicts have histories of criminal arrests. In addition, many addicts have a history of multiple arrests. Overall, according to one survey, the average number of arrests among heroin addicts is two for every three years between age eighteen and entry into treatment.[9] These figures most likely reflect the fact that (1) addicts belong to a subculture in which illegal activity is a common practice—this point is further substantiated by the finding that many addicts had criminal histories *before* the onset of addiction; (2) the drug habit requires substantial amounts of money and often the addict turns to crime to obtain these funds; and (3) narcotics use itself involves frequent violation of laws against possession and sales of narcotics so that even a person having no prior record of criminal behavior will not be able to avoid criminal activities after a period of time as an addict.

As implied in the preceding paragraph, the answer to the second question—that is, whether heroin use leads to criminal behavior—would seem to be that it does only in the case of a small percentage of addicts; a large proportion of addicts will have already had a criminal history before the onset of addiction. However, there seems to be a direct relationship between continued use of heroin and increased criminal activity, most likely because addicts need funds to buy narcotics. Some support for this statement can be found in the fact that when the retail price of heroin went up in New York City, a rise in crime rates soon followed.[10] Furthermore, the types of crimes that were on the increase were those specifically related to obtaining money—for example, robbery, larceny, and auto theft—whereas the incidence of other crimes, such as manslaughter and rape, remained about the same.

Other Opiates

Heroin is only one of several opium derivatives that are commonly abused. Among these substances are morphine, opium, and codeine. These drugs are natural opiates. There are also a number of chemically related substances called synthetic narcotics, which are not naturally occurring but are made by laboratory methods. The natural opiates will be briefly discussed first.

Opium

Opium is the first substance obtained in the production of opium narcotics. This substance contains morphine and codeine as well as other narcotic compounds. (As noted earlier in the chapter, heroin is produced from morphine by a chemical process.) In many parts of the world, especially in the Middle and Far East, the use of opium (which is eaten or smoked) has been a common practice for hundreds of years. At one time opium was widely used in this country, but this is no longer true today.

Opium has been medicinally used in two forms: (1) *laudanum* (tincture of opium) which contains 10 percent opium in a water and alcohol solution; and

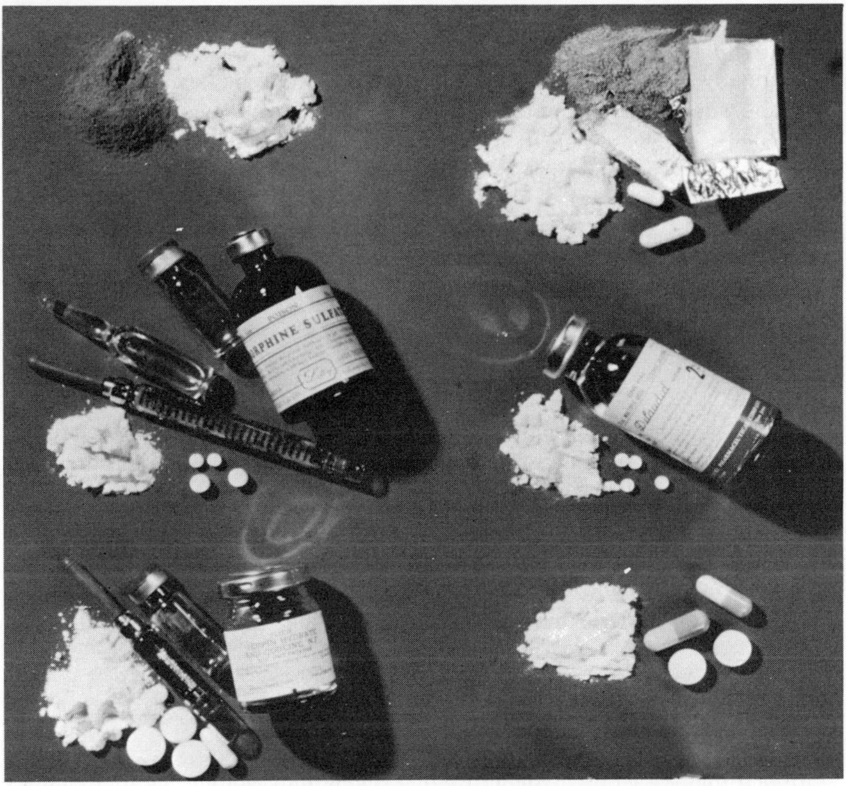

SOURCE: Drug Enforcement Administration, U.S. Department of Justice

Figure 2. The many forms of opiates. Opium derivatives may be found in forms ranging from heroin as a fine white or brown powder as it is sold on the street in capsules, glassine envelopes or foil to the medical preparations of morphine sulfate which come packaged in bottles, vials, and ampules, as well as in tablet form. Many hospitals now use glass containers fitted with needles which, with plunger attached, can be directly used for injection. Dilaudid, or hydromorphone, is a semisynthetic derivative of morphine, while codeine is naturally occurring.

(2) *paregoric,* which in addition to opium, alcohol and water, contains camphor, benzoic acid, and anise oil. Only the latter mixture is still available today. It is sometimes used by heroin addicts when heroin is not available, although a small number of paregoric addicts do exist.

Morphine

Morphine is of course the active ingredient of heroin, and differs from it only slightly—the most important difference to the addict is that when heroin is injected, its onset of effects is more rapid than that of morphine. The effects of morphine last somewhat longer, however, than do those of heroin, and when morphine is used as an analgesic it is only half as potent as the same amount (by weight) of heroin.

Originally widely dispensed in this country before the turn of the century, morphine was seen as the preferred form of treatment for many different medical problems, and was freely dispensed by physicians. It has even been used as a treatment for alcoholism, a practice which lasted well into this century.

Addiction to morphine, in contrast to addiction to heroin, usually occurs as a consequence of a course of medical treatment during which the drug is taken regularly to relieve pain. Addiction may also be seen in doctors or nurses to whom the drug is relatively accessible.

Codeine

Codeine is another active ingredient in opium. Its effects are very similar to those of morphine, although it is considerably less potent than morphine and therefore a correspondingly larger dose is required to produce the same effects. It is a common ingredient of cough medicine, and is also useful in relieving pain, as are all the opiates. It is generally abused only when other, more potent opiates are not available.

Among the *synthetic* narcotics, meperidine and methadone are the best known.

Meperidine

Meperidine (Demerol, Dolantin, and Dolantol are among the trade names for this drug), like so many of the synthetic narcotics, has received wide usage because it was believed to have many of the positive analgesic qualities of morphine, but few of the undesirable side effects. As has been the case for many of the synthetic narcotics, it proved to be just as addicting as the naturally occurring opiates. Next to morphine, meperidine is one of the most widely used narcotic analgesics in medical practice. For this reason, as well as the mistaken belief that it was less addicting, many health personnel to whom it was available began using it regularly and subsequently became addicted to it.

Methadone

Methadone, also known under the trade names Amidone, Diadone, Dolophine, and Methadon, among others, is a synthetic narcotic analgesic best known for its wide use in the treatment of heroin addiction. Having pain-relieving qualities similar to those possessed by morphine, methadone was originally used as a narcotic analgesic, and has addiction potential itself. Today, however, it is primarily used in the treatment of heroin addiction because it blocks the euphoric effects produced by heroin. (See Chapter 8 for a discussion of this use of methadone.)

Notes

1. J. A. O'Donnell, *Narcotic Addicts in Kentucky* (Washington, D.C.: U.S. Public Health Service Publication No. 1881, 1969), pp. 23–30.
2. J. D. Sapira, J. C. Ball, and H. Penn, "Causes of Death Among Institutionalized Narcotic Addicts," in J. C. Ball and C. D. Chambers, eds., *The Epidemiology of Heroin Addiction in the United States*. (Springfield, Ill.: Thomas, 1970), pp. 251–262.
3. A. R. Lindesmith, *Opiate Addiction* (Bloomington, Ind.: Principia Press, 1947).
4. H. Blumberg et al, "British Opiate Users: II. Differences Between Those Given an Opiate Script and Those Not Given One," *International Journal of the Addictions* 9 (1974): pp. 205–220.
5. J. M. Scher, "The Impact of the Drug Abuser on the Work Organization," in J. M. Scher. ed., *Drug Abuse in Industry* (Springfield, Ill.: Thomas, 1973), pp. 5–16.
6. P. J. Bourne, "Issues in Addiction," in P. J. Bourne, ed., *Addiction* (New York: Academic Press, 1974), pp. 1–19.
7. J. C. Ball and C. D. Chambers, eds., *The Epidemiology of Opiate Addiction in the United States* (Springfield, Ill.: Thomas, 1970), pp. 5–21.
8. C. Winick, "Epidemiology of Narcotics Use," in D. M. Wilner and G. G. Kassebaum, eds., *Narcotics* (New York: McGraw-Hill, 1965), pp. 3–18.
9. G. Nash, *The Impact of Drug Abuse Treatment upon Criminality: A Look at 19 Programs* (A summary version) (Montclair, N.J.: Montclair State College, 1973), p. 1.2.
10. G. F. Brown and L. P. Silverman, "The Retail Price of Heroin: Estimation and Applications," *Journal of the American Statistical Association* 69 (1974): pp. 595–606.

Selected Bibliography

Abel, E. L. *Drugs and Behavior: A Primer in Neuropsychopharmacology*. New York: Wiley, 1974.

Ausubel, D. P. *Drug Addiction: Physiological, Psychological, and Sociological Aspects*. New York: Random House, 1958, 1964.

Bourne, P. J., ed. *Addiction*. New York: Academic Press, 1974.

Brecher, E. M. *Licit and Illicit Drugs*. Boston: Little, Brown, 1972.

Bucky, S. F. "The Relationship Between Background and Extent of Heroin Use," *American Journal of Psychiatry* 130 (1973): 709–710.

Chein, I.; Gerard, D. L.; Lee, R. S.; and Rosenfield, E. *The Road to H: Narcotics, Delinquency, and Social Policy*, New York: Basic Books, 1964.

Cherubin, C. E., "The Medical Sequelae of Narcotic Addiction." *Annals of Internal Medicine* 67 (1967): 23–33.

Cimino, J. A.; Doud, R. M.; Andima, H. S.; and West, S. A. "Narcotic Addiction in the United States: A Nationwide Survey." *Contemporary Drug Problems* 2 (1973): 401–415.

Cushman, P. "Narcotic Addiction and Crime." *Rhode Island Medical Journal* 57 (1974): 197–204.

Drug Abuse Council, *Heroin Maintenance: The Issues*. Washington, D.C.: Drug Abuse Council, 1973.

Fink, M.; Zaks, A.; Resnick, R.; and Freedman, A. "Treatment of Heroin Dependence with Opiate Antagonists." In Masserman, J. H., ed. *Handbook of Psychiatric Therapies, New York: Science House, 1966*.

Hofmann, F. G. *A Handbook on Drug and Alcohol Abuse*. New York: Oxford, 1975.

Huberty, D. J. "Civil Commitment of the Narcotic Addict: Evaluation of a Treatment Model," *Crime and Delinquency* 18 (1972): 99–109.

Jaffe, J. H. "Drug Addiction and Drug Abuse." In Goodman, L. S., and Gilman, A. *The Pharmacological Basis of Therapeutics*. 4th ed. New York: Macmillan, 1970.

Jaffe, J. H. "Narcotic Analgesics." In Goodman, L. S., and Gilman, A. *The Pharmacological Basis of Therapeutics,* 4th ed. New York: Macmillan, 1970.

Kozel, N. J.; Dupont, R. L; and Brown, B. S. "Narcotics and Crime: A Study of Narcotic Involvement in an Offender Population." *International Journal of the Addictions* 7 (1972): 443–450.

Louria, D. B.; Hensle, T.; and Rose, J. "The Major Medical Complications of Heroin Addiction." *Annals of Internal Medicine* 67 (1967): 1–22.

Markott, E. L. "Synanon in Drug Addiction." In Masserman, J. H., ed. *Handbook of Psychiatric Therapies*. New York: Science House, 1966.

National Clearinghouse for Drug Abuse Information. *Narcotic Antagonists,* Report Series 26, No. 1, 1973.

National Clearinghouse for Drug Abuse Information. *Methadone: The Drug and Its Therapeutic Uses in the Treatment of Addiction,* Report Series 31, No. 1, 1974.

Newman, R. G.; Bashkow, S.; and Cates, M. "Arrest Histories Before and After Admission to a Methadone Maintenance Treatment Program," *Contemporary Drug Problems* 2 (1973): 417–430.

Platt, J. J., and Labate, C. *Heroin Addiction: Theory, Research, and Treatment*. New York: Wiley-Interscience, 1976.

Platt, J. J.; Scura, W. C.; and Hannon, J. "Problem-solving Thinking of Youthful Incarcerated Heroin Addicts." *Journal of Community Psychology* 1 (1973): 278–281.

Platt, J. J.; Scura, W. C.; and Hoffman, A. "Heroin Addiction Incidence Among Youthful Offenders, 1968–1972." *Journal of Community Psychology* 1 (1973): 408–411.

Ray, O. S. *Drugs, Society, and Human Behavior*. St. Louis: Mosby, 1972.

Richter, R. W., ed. *Medical Aspects of Drug Abuse*. Hagerstown, Md.: Harper & Row, 1975.

Singh, J. M.; Miller, L.; and Lal, H. *Drug Addiction: Clinical and Socio-legal Aspects,* Vol. 2. Mt. Kisco, N.Y.: Futura, 1972.

Steinberg, H., ed. *Scientific Basis of Drug Dependence*. London: Churchill, 1969.

Wikler, A., ed. *The Addictive States*. Baltimore: Williams and Wilkins, 1968.

Chapter 5

Cannabis: Marijuana and Hashish

Like so many other common drugs of abuse, both marijuana and hashish have a long and colorful history. Over 4,500 years ago, marijuana was referred to by the Chinese Emperor Shen Nung, who recommended it as a useful remedy for such problems as rheumatism, malaria, constipation, and absentmindedness. But the Chinese were not the only people in the ancient world to use cannabis. Also using it for a variety of purposes were the Indians, the Arabs, and the Ancient Greeks. In fact, the first marijuana "epidemic" is said to have occurred in North Africa almost 1,000 years ago.

Marijuana is one of the best-known and most widely used drugs in this country today. A number of surveys have illustrated just how widely used marijuana actually is. The estimate most often heard is that about four out of every ten young Americans have tried marijuana. A survey conducted by the National Commission on Marijuana and Drug Abuse in 1972 estimated that at least 24 million Americans over the age of eleven had experimented with marijuana, and that some 8.3 million of these were using the drug at the time of the survey. It has been estimated that some 200 million people throughout the world are currently using marijuana.[1]

What Is Marijuana?

Marijuana comes from the hemp plant *Cannabis sativa,* the fibers of which have been used for many years to produce rope, twine, and cord. The hemp plant grows widely throughout the world, in both tropical and temperate climates. At its maximum growth, it can reach a height of fifteen to twenty feet. It should be noted that there are several major variations of the hemp plant. One variation which has been cultivated primarily for use in producing fiber, contains relatively little of the resin, from which the active ingredient is taken. Another variation is grown primarily for its resin. The fiber type is usually found growing wild in the United States. The variations containing the greatest amounts of psychoactive substance come from India, Mexico, Jamaica, and

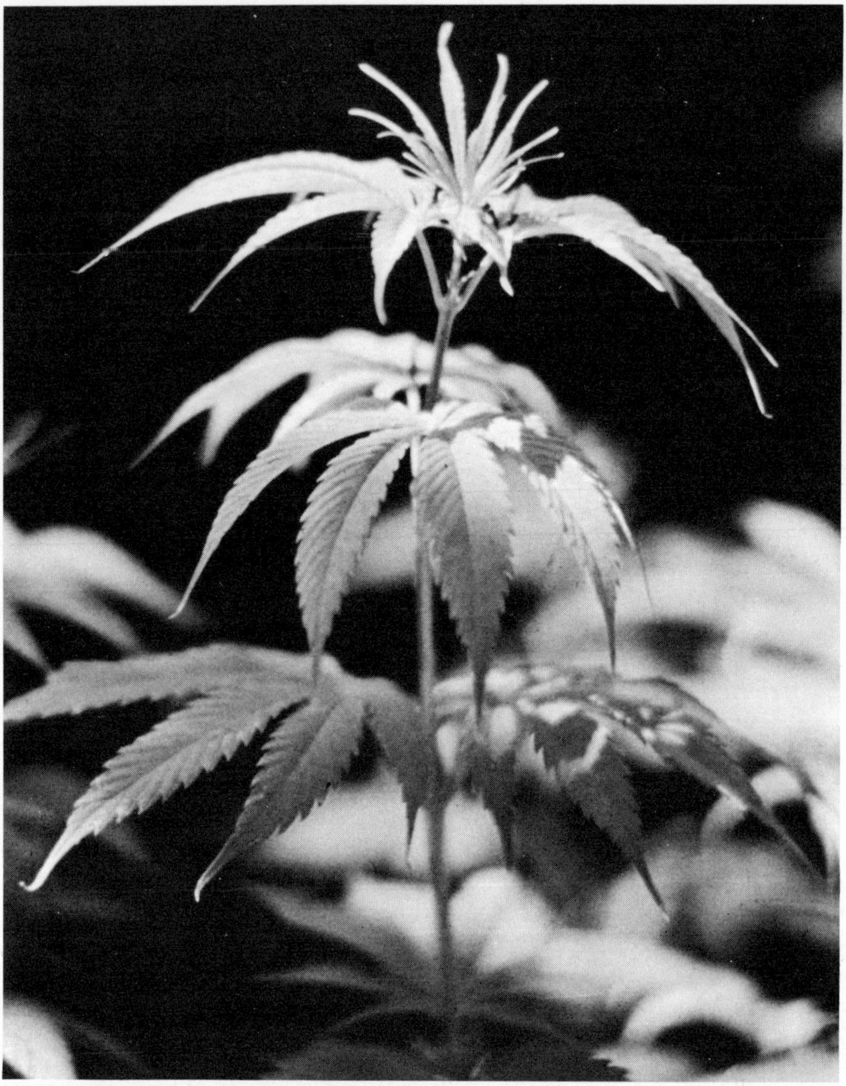

SOURCE: Drug Enforcement Administration, U.S. Department of Justice
Figure 3. This close-up of Cannabis sativa, *the marijuana plant, illustrates its characteristically serrated leaves, as well as the flowering top of the plant. Overall, the plant may reach a height of 15 to 20 feet.*

North Africa. The seeds of this plant have also been used as feed for poultry, and when crushed, in paint to speed its drying, and as soap. But the part of the plant in which we are interested is the sticky yellow resin which is found mainly in the flowering top of the female plant and the surrounding leaves. It is also found, though to a lesser degree, in the lower parts of the plant, from which rope

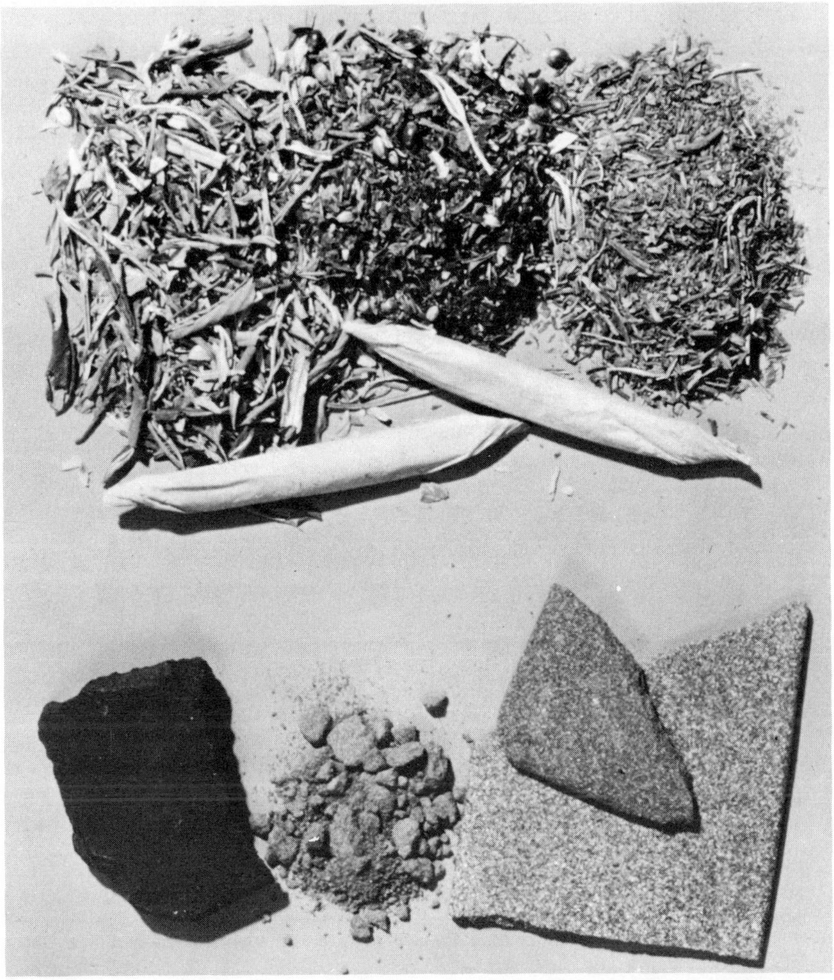

SOURCE: Drug Enforcement Administration, U.S. Department of Justice
Figure 4. Marijuana and hashish. Marijuana usually consists of the dried, chopped flowering tops, leaves, and stems of the cannabis plant, even though the most potent marijuana is made only from the flowering tops of the female plant. Hashish, scraped from cannabis leaves or obtained by boiling them, is generally sold in compressed brick form.

is made. The resin, which is secreted by and covers the tops of the plants and leaves, is known as *hashish* or *hash* in this country and as *charas* in India. It may be scraped from the leaves, or obtained by boiling those parts of the plant it covers. Hashish is perhaps six or seven times as potent as marijuana, which is obtained by drying the flowering tops, leaves, and stems of the *Cannabis sativa* plant. Marijuana is less potent because of the lower concentration of resin in the leaves and stems.

Only recently have scientists been able to isolate and study the major chemical compound in cannabis which is responsible for its psychoactive effects. It is now known that cannabis contains more than twenty unique chemical compounds, only two of which have hallucinogenic properties. Interestingly, while most of the other compounds have no biological effects, a few have the ability to destroy bacteria or to produce sedation.

The active ingredient in marijuana and hashish was first isolated in the 1960s. This substance, which is a complex molecule known as tetrahydrocannabinol (THC), comprises approximately 0.05 to 8 percent of the total content of marijuana. By contrast, hashish may contain from 5 to 12 percent THC. Jamaican ganga, made primarily from the flowering tops and small leaves, may have a THC content of 4 to 8 percent. Table 5.1 shows the THC content of the various types of hashish and marijuana available on the American market. For legal purposes both marijuana and hashish are often described in terms of their THC content.

TABLE 5.1 CONTENT OF THC, BY WEIGHT, IN MARIJUANA AND HASHISH FROM VARIOUS SOURCES

SOURCE	PERCENTAGE OF THC (BY WEIGHT)
Marijuana	
United States	Less than two-tenths of 1 percent
Mexico	Less than 1 percent
Jamaica and Southeast Asia	2 to 4 percent
Ganga	
Jamaica	4 to 8 percent
India	Less than Jamaican
Hashish (Charas)	
India	5 to 12 percent

SOURCE: *Marijuana: A Signal of Misunderstanding.* First Report of the National Commission on Marijuana and Drug Abuse (Washington, D.C.: U.S. Government Printing Office, 1972).

How Marijuana Is Used

In this country marijuana and hashish are most commonly smoked in cigarette form. Pipe smoking of these drugs, seen less often in this country than cigarette smoking, is more commonly practiced in the Middle East. Both marijuana and hashish can either be smoked alone or mixed with cigarette or pipe tobacco. As with many other illegal drugs, the user rarely knows the actual THC content of the marijuana being smoked, or even what the other ingredients may be. Actually, smoking is a relatively inefficient way of getting THC into the smoker's bloodstream. This is because a large amount of the smoke containing the drug may escape into the air; in addition, the THC itself may be destroyed by the heat of a burning cigarette. One recent study suggested that

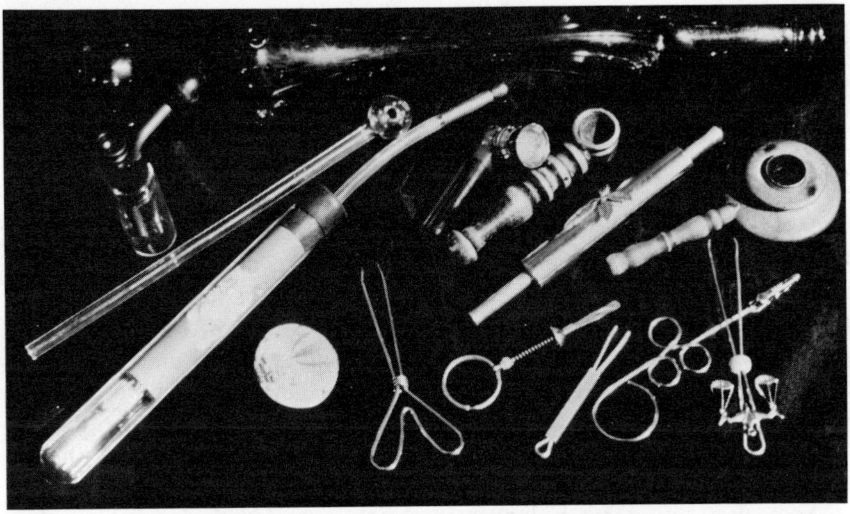

SOURCE: Drug Enforcement Administration, U.S. Department of Justice
Figure 5. The paraphernalia of cannabis abuse includes pipes of varying designs, usually with relatively small bowls, as well as hookahs. Various kinds of cigarette holders are also illustrated. All of these are designed to obtain the maximum number of puffs from small butts (''roaches''). For this reason they are called ''roach holders.''

only about 50 percent of the THC in a typical marijuana cigarette will actually reach the smoker's bloodstream, but the actual percentage may vary from 20 to 80 percent. When the drug is smoked, however, its effects are produced almost immediately. The amount of time required for the effects to be felt may range from a few seconds to a few minutes at the most. Thus, the major characteristics of smoking the drug are (1) relatively inefficient delivery to the bloodstream; and (2) rapidly felt effects of maximum strength and minimum duration.

Another form of administration involves injecting the resin directly into the veins. Obviously, this method, depending upon the THC concentration of the drug being used, produces a very different type of high than that produced by other methods of administration.

Cannabis products may also be added to food or beverages—for example, they may be added to baked products or brewed in tea. Naturally, this form of administration results in a slower uptake of the drug by the body, depending both upon the type and amount of food already present in the stomach, as well as the food ingested along with the drug. Administration of the drug by this method usually results in a weaker but more prolonged effect.

Length of Effect

One factor which seems to influence the duration of the effects of marijuana or hashish is the amount of prior exposure to these drugs. Persons who have had considerable experience with cannabis tend to metabolize it more rapidly, and perhaps even differently, than do individuals with little or no experience. The way in which marijuana is metabolized is important because it is through this process that the effects of the drug are activated. Later on, this same process helps deactivate the effects just prior to the removal of the drug from the body.

Tolerance

Whether or not a person develops a tolerance to marijuana and hashish seems to depend upon the pattern and extent of use. It appears that when high doses of these drugs are used regularly, for extended periods of time, psychological tolerance may develop. However, tolerance also develops to the unpleasant physical side effects of the drug, so that the long-term user may experience fewer such side effects than the newly initiated one, and may be able to function quite normally while intoxicated. In both light and moderate usage, the development of tolerance is minimal, although the "high" may have a shorter duration.

Some users report that the longer they smoke cannabis, the less they need on subsequent occasions to obtain the same effects. This phenomenon, called *reverse tolerance,* may be the result of one or more of the following: (1) changes in the body's capacity to convert the drug to an active chemical; (2) learning how to consciously maximize the effects of the drug; or (3) the development of an ability to recognize the subtle cues of intoxication at low doses of the drug.

Of course it should also be recognized that the effects of any drug may be different for different individuals, since each person has unique personality traits as well as different expectations for the drug experience. Likewise, the setting in which a person takes a drug may influence the effects it has. Also, in contrast to a drug such as alcohol, people find that it is easier to suppress some of the effects of a marijuana high.

Pattern of Use

The National Commission on Marijuana and Drug Abuse reported that there are five general patterns of marijuana use. Each of these patterns is associated with certain personality traits, and is characteristic of a particular type of marijuana user. These will be briefly described below.

Experimental users. Experimental users comprise the largest number of users. This group consists of individuals who have tried marijuana but who either have not continued to use it or who use it rarely. (This group represents 41 percent of adults over eighteen and 45 percent of young people between the ages of twelve and seventeen.) Persons in this group appear to differ very little from nonusers with regard to personality, achievement in school, occupation, social adjustment, and overall life-style. Their initial reasons for using the drug were related to curiosity and a desire to share the experience of others.

Intermittent users. Intermittent users include individuals who use marijuana on an average of two to four times a month. This group represents some 12 percent of adults and 19 percent of young people aged twelve to seventeen who have ever tried the drug. Persons belonging to this group tend to use marijuana only within a social context; use of the drug is clearly linked to social occasions for the purpose of relaxation and recreation, such as listening to music, watching television, and eating. Persons in this group tend to have similar initial motivations for using the drug, and are likely to be somewhat liberal and concerned with personal growth, expression, and independence.

Moderate and heavy users. Moderate and heavy users comprise the smallest group, accounting for some 8 percent of adults and 9 percent of youths. Moderate and heavy users may use marijuana from several times weekly to several times daily, perhaps smoking as many as five cigarettes on a single occasion. The moderate users are highly similar to those in the intermittent group, and tend to use marijuana for the same reasons as the intermittent users. Likewise, heavy users may have started using marijuana for the same reason, but may also use it for "kicks," to "expand their awareness," or to escape from boredom or anxiety. Heavy users tend to be rather unhappy, immature, pleasure-seeking individuals who are generally unconcerned with the rules by which the rest of society lives. One study found that although individuals in this group were intellectually bright, they were nonetheless underachievers who were generally not living up to their potential. Many of them were college dropouts who also had poor work histories. It was also found that heavy users more often came from broken homes or had histories of alcohol or drug problems than did the intermittent users; in addition, many individuals in this group came from a lower socioeconomic background. For heavy users, marijuana smoking, while often carried out in a group setting, was not done primarily as a social activity but for the personal effects of the drug.

Very heavy users. Very heavy users include individuals for whom marijuana use and intoxication are almost continuous. It is very much smaller in size than the other groups, and is characterized by psychological dependence on marijuana, lethargy, lack of interest in activities other than those related to drug use, and a decrease in level of social functioning. This group also tends to prefer hashish over marijuana because of the former's greater potency.

Characteristics of Marijuana Users

Because marijuana use in this country is extremely widespread, cutting across all levels of society, it is difficult to develop an accurate picture of the "typical" marijuana user. However, it is possible to identify a number of characteristics which seem to be shared by a large percentage of these individuals. (These characteristics are based on the findings of a survey conducted by the National Commission on Marijuana and Drug Abuse.)

Sex. Although there was a time when almost twice as many males as females were using marijuana, today a greater proportion of females have begun using the drug. In fact, in some groups of young people there are as many female users as there are male users.

Race and Religion. Marijuana use today appears to be almost equally distributed among racial and religious groups. There does, however, appear to be a slightly higher rate of usage among Catholics and Jews than among Protestants. More frequent use by the former groups may be related to the fact that use is higher in urban and suburban areas, where the largest Catholic and Jewish populations are found.

Geographic Distribution. There is a disproportionate geographic distribution of marijuana use in this country. Rates of usage have been found to be higher in the northeastern and western states than in the north central and southern states.

Socioeconomic Status. Marijuana use appears to be more prevalent among individuals earning above-average incomes, although the drug is also used by members of the lower and middle income groups. Use appears to be fairly evenly distributed among such occupational groups as salespeople, clerical workers, and skilled, semiskilled, and unskilled workers.

Education. Marijuana use appears to be more prevalent among college-educated individuals than among individuals with less education. The highest rates of use are found among persons who have attended—if not completed—college. The next highest rates of use are found among college graduates, followed by high-school graduates, and individuals who have had some high-school education. Finally, the lowest rates of use occur among individuals having an eighth-grade education or less. The commission found that whereas 21 percent of the college graduates surveyed had experimented with marijuana, only 5 percent of those with less than an eighth-grade education had ever been exposed to it.

Age. The greatest amount of marijuana use is among young people eighteen to twenty-one years of age; the least amount of use is among those over fifty years of age.[2]

Effects of Marijuana

The physical effects of marijuana are minimal, and may or may not be present in all individuals who use it (see Table 5.2). This reflects the fact that marijuana primarily affects psychological functioning. Use of low-to-moderate doses of marijuana may result in some or all of the changes that are described in Table 5.2.

TABLE 5.2 EFFECTS OF MARIJUANA ON THE BODY

BODILY FUNCTION OR ORGAN	EFFECT
Nervous System—General	1. Increased amounts of time may be spent in sleeping and dreaming.
Nervous System—The Eye	1. Reddening of the conjunctiva. 2. Pupil size may decrease slightly. 3. Rapid side-to-side movement (nystagmus) of the eyeball may occur.
Respiratory System	1. No change in breathing for cigarette smokers; nonsmokers may show some decrease in respiratory functioning. 2. Coughing may result from the irritant effects of the smoke.
Circulatory System	1. Pulse rate may increase slightly. 2. Blood pressure may decrease slightly upon standing, and increase upon reclining.
Musculature	1. Slight decrease in muscular strength may occur. 2. Slight hand tremor may occur.
Other	1. Dryness of the mouth. 2. Possible increase in appetite; often a craving for sweets. 3. Slight decrease in body temperature.

SOURCE: J. H. Mendelson, A. M. Rossi, and R. E. Meyer, eds., *The Use of Marijuana: A Psychological and Physiological Inquiry* (New York: Plenum, 1974).

Desired Reactions

One of the best descriptions of the subjective effects of marijuana smoking is the one that was offered by Dr. Jesse L. Steinfeld, Surgeon General of the U.S. Public Health Service, in his testimony before the House Select Committee on Crime.

> The onset of action after smoking is within 10 to 20 minutes, and the effects may persist for 3 hours. The psychic effects generally begin with a feeling of relaxation and detachment. Audio-visual sensations are intensified, with color perceptions often the most affected. Time perception is altered, usually manifested by a slowing of subjective time.
>
> Emotions are loosened, with euphoria* being more common than dysphoria. Inappropriate laughing jags or crying spells have been described, while anxiety and feelings of suspiciousness are rare. Thought is dreamlike and fantasy-laden, but the person can pull himself together when necessary and perform adequately.

*Euphoria refers to a state of well being or elation. Dysphoria refers to a state characterized by feeling unwell or unhappy.

> Some individuals experience drowsiness and feelings of hunger; others feel unable to communicate properly.
>
> The individual is often passive and withdrawn. However, as with all disinhibiting agents, he might behave in an unrestrained, emotional manner. While marijuana does not possess aphrodisiac properties, the prolongation of subjective time may alter the perception of an erotic experience.[3]

Other symptoms which may occur include a decrease in hearing acuity, an initial feeling of friendliness, which later decreases, and a decrease in aggressiveness.

Of course, the extent to which the individual experiences these effects depends upon such factors as the dose taken, the ability of the user's body to absorb the drug, the amount of prior experience with the drug, as well as the personality of the user and his or her overall adjustment. Thus, not all persons who use marijuana will experience these effects, and those who do will not always find them pleasurable. In fact, some users may find them very unpleasant, and may not use the drug again. In one study, marijuana users who were asked to compare the effects of marijuana with those of alcohol expressed an almost unanimous preference for marijuana.[4] Among their reasons for choosing it they cited the fact that with marijuana there is less change in perception and fewer unpleasant body sensations as well as a greater feeling of control. Interestingly, the subjects in this study, all of whom were experienced marijuana users (which may have biased some of the reported preferences), felt that alcohol was a more effective reducer of inhibitions and for this reason they preferred it over marijuana in large social gatherings.

Adverse Reactions

The use of marijuana may produce unpleasant reactions in even the most experienced user, but, generally speaking, these reactions tend to occur infrequently. When they do occur, they may take the form of feelings of anxiety, depression, suspiciousness, panic, fatigue, and loss of memory. Delusional thinking may also be present, as well as dizziness, nausea, and incoordination. In rare instances, a loss of cognitive controls may take place, resulting in a state of panic, which could lead the individual to injure himself or others.

As mentioned above, adverse reactions tend to be relatively rare for users of marijuana, compared to users of other psychoactive drugs, such as LSD. And generally the intensity of these reactions will decrease with the passage of time, during which the individual sleeps or is "talked down" from the high by companions. Of course, the drug is being metabolized during this time, so that it is gradually being removed from the user's body.

A user who is severely psychologically disturbed may find that using the drug in heavy doses could trigger a psychotic episode, which might last a few days, and occasionally even require brief hospitalization. It is not known, however, whether such reactions can occur in persons who do not have preexisting psychiatric illness.

Although studies have shown that few long-term physical abnormalities can be attributed to marijuana use, it has been suggested that prolonged use of the drug may result in brain damage, or at least a decrease in brain functioning. Here again, there is insufficient evidence at the present time to make a definitive statement regarding this issue.

There does seem to be some evidence suggesting that long-term, heavy usage of marijuana may lead to certain psychological changes, including decreased motivation and an inability to function normally in society and to interact with others. The individual who exhibits this syndrome may "drop out" and lose interest in almost all activities other than those related to using marijuana. Such reactions are not always the direct result of drug use, however, but are more often related to the individual's lack of direction prior to becoming a user; in addition, their behavior may reflect the attitudes and mores of the drug culture.

Marijuana Use and Driving

One of the most important questions for the law enforcement officer is whether marijuana use can interfere with a person's ability to operate a motor vehicle—for example, as alcohol does. The answer to this question is simply not known at the present time. On the one hand, we do know that marijuana use can adversely affect some of the skills necessary for safely operating a car—such as the sense of time and the ability to make complex judgments. On the other hand, the amount of the drug taken is usually small and some degree of conscious control over its effects can be exercised. To further complicate the picture, a great deal depends on whether the user is an experienced marijuana smoker, whether the user is also taking other drugs such as tranquilizers, alcohol, or psychedelic substances, and, of course, the actual THC content of the cigarettes smoked. In one of the most widely known studies on this subject, Dr. A. Crancer found the effects of alcohol upon driving ability to be greater than those of marijuana. However, while considerably more research is needed before a definitive answer to this question can be reached, one must question how the skills required by such a complex activity as driving can fail to be affected by blood concentrations of THC which are equal in effect to intoxicating doses of alcohol.

Is Marijuana Addicting?

Contrary to popular belief, physical withdrawal symptoms do not follow the discontinuation of marijuana use as they do in the case of heroin. This is because marijuana is *not* physically addicting, and physiological dependence does not occur. On the other hand, psychological dependence to marijuana may develop in habitual heavy users. In the case of some heavy users of marijuana, restlessness and anxiety may develop upon cessation of smoking, but these symptoms are not different from those seen in tobacco smokers who have gone "cold turkey."

Marijuana Use and Criminal Behavior

It was once widely believed that marijuana use, by weakening self-control, increasing aggressive tendencies, impairing judgment, and decreasing the sense of individual responsibility, led to criminal behavior. This is not believed to be true by most experts in the field today, and the overwhelming weight of available evidence tends to support this view. The National Commission on Marijuana and Drug Abuse, in summarizing its own and prior research on the subject, reached the following conclusions.

With respect to crimes involving violence:

1. Marijuana decreases the acting out of aggressive impulses by calming the user, interfering with muscular coordination and decreasing motor activity, and producing lethargy.
2. Individuals who are arrested for marijuana-related offenses tend *not* to have been arrested for violent crimes.
3. When offenders who use marijuana are compared with those who do not, the latter group is found to have been arrested or convicted more often for such violent crimes as murder, forcible rape, aggravated assault, and armed robbery.
4. Marijuana use was no more frequent prior to the commission of an offense in which violence occurred than in which violence did not occur. (Interestingly, alcohol was used more often prior to the commission of an offense in which violence occurred.)

With respect to nonviolent crime:

1. There is no evidence to indicate that marijuana users, even heavy users, commit crimes to obtain funds to purchase the drug as do many heroin users.
2. Few marijuana users (less than 10 percent in one study) who are arrested have prior arrests for offenses such as assault, robbery, burglary, or larceny.[5]

It is true, however—and this may appear to be contradictory at first—that there is a definite statistical correlation between marijuana use and criminal behavior. This finding simply reflects the fact that many users come from the same "high-risk" populations in which crimes and delinquent behavior are most likely to occur. Thus, there was a strong likelihood that these individuals would commit crimes whether or not they used marijuana. Thus the correlation between criminal behavior and marijuana use is only coincidental. The fact is that both activities reflect a number of other factors, including socioeconomic background, low income, and so forth. Clearly, then, it would be inaccurate to conclude that marijuana use itself leads to criminal behavior.

The Sale of Marijuana

The sale of marijuana, like that of most other illegal drugs, has a fantastically large profit potential. Richard Callahan, regional director of the Bureau of Narcotics and Dangerous Drugs, testified in 1970 before the House Select Committee on Crime that a one kilogram brick of marijuana (2.2 pounds), which could be purchased in some parts of Mexico for $15 to $20, would be resalable on the United States side of the border for $50 to $75. The kilogram of marijuana could be made into some 2,500 cigarettes, each retailing for one dollar, and result in a profit of nearly $2,500. Callahan estimated that a good-sized marijuana operation could have an earning capacity of $100,000 a year.

Marijuana and Other Drug Use

Does marijuana use lead to the use of narcotics such as heroin? Research conducted to answer this question indicates that whereas most heroin users have used marijuana at one time or another, only a small proportion of marijuana users ever uses heroin. One recent survey of the research on this issue reports on several studies which found that a very large number of heroin users had smoked marijuana prior to using heroin.[6] Another recent study suggested that the use of marijuana "is a crucial stage prior to the use of other illicit drugs, such as LSD, pills, or heroin." Furthermore, it was found that "only 2 to 3 percent of . . . legal drug users [in this study] progress directly to these other illicit drugs without first trying marijuana."[7] Yet in none of the studies surveyed was there evidence to allow one to conclude that marijuana use in itself leads to heroin use. Rather, it appears that marijuana use is simply one step in a progression from legal drugs, such as cigarettes and alcoholic beverages, to marijuana to other illicit drugs.

As stated above, most heroin users have used marijuana, but this finding simply reflects the fact that marijuana is typically the first illicit drug used by high school-age youth; thus it is used by individuals who go on to use narcotics as well as by those who do not. What is significant is that heavy marijuana users may have fewer reservations about using illegal drugs in general, and thus may be more likely to experiment with a wide variety of drugs, including heroin, than nonusers. Generally speaking, however, there is no conclusive evidence to date to suggest that marijuana use eventually leads to the use of heroin, and there appears to be nothing in marijuana itself which would necessitate the use of stronger drugs.

Notes

1. L. E. Hollister, "Marijuana in Man: Three Years Later," *Science* 172 (1971): pp. 21–29.
2. *Marijuana: A Signal of Misunderstanding*. First Report of the National Commission on Marijuana and Drug Abuse (Washington, D.C.: U.S. Government Printing Office, 1972), pp. 71–76.
3. *Marijuana*. First Report by the Select Committee on Crime (Washington D.C.: U.S. Government Printing Office, 1970), pp. 4–5.
4. C. Tart, *On Being Stoned* (Palo Alto, Calif.: Science and Behavior Press, 1971), p. 47.
5. *Marijuana: A Signal of Misunderstanding*, pp. 71–76.
6. J. J. Platt and C. Labate, *Heroin Addiction: Theory, Research, and Treatment* (New York: Wiley-Interscience, 1976), pp. 183–184.
7. D. Kandel, "Stages in Adolescent Involvement in Drug Use," *Science* 190 (1975): pp. 912–913.

Selected Bibliography

Brecher, E. M. *Licit and Illicit Drugs*. Boston: Little, Brown, 1972.

Campbell, A. M.; Evans, M.; Thomson, L. G.; and Williams, M. J. "Cerebral Atrophy in Young Cannabis Smokers." *Lancet* 2 (1971): 1219 ff.

Crancer, A., Jr.; Dille, J. M.; Delay, J. C.; Wallace, J. E.; and Haykin, M. D. "Comparison of the Effects of Marijuana on Simulated Driving Performance." *Science* 164 (1969): 851 ff.

Hofmann, F. G. *A Handbook on Drug and Alcohol Abuse*. New York: Oxford, 1975.

Hollister, L. E. "Clinical Pharmacology of Hallucinogens and Marijuana." In Zarafonetis, C. J., ed. *Drug Abuse: Proceedings of the International Conference*. Philadelphia: Lea/Febiger, 1972.

Jaffe, J. "Drug Addiction and Drug Abuse." In Goodman, L., and Gilman, A, eds. *The Pharmacological Basis of Therapeutics*, 4th ed. New York: Macmillan, 1970.

Leavitt, F. *Drugs and Behavior*. Philadelphia: Saunders, 1974.

Low, M. D.; Klonoff, H.; and Marcus, A. "The Neurophysiological Basis of the Marijuana Experience." *Canadian Medical Association Journal* 108 (1973): 157–165.

Mechoulam, R. "Marijuana Chemistry." *Science* 168 (1970): 1159–1166.

Mendelson, J. H.; Rossi, A. M.; and Meyer, R. E., eds. *The Use of Marihuana: A Psychological and Physiological Inquiry*. New York: Plenum, 1974.

Pillard, R. C. "Marijuana." *New England Journal of Medicine* 283 (1970): 294–303.

Schultes, R. E. "Hallucinogens of Plant Origin." *Science* 163 (1969): 245–254.

Weil, A. T. "Adverse Reactions to Marihuana." *New England Journal of Medicine* 282 (1970): 997 ff.

Weil, A. T.; Zinberg, N. E.; and Nelson, J. M. "Clinical and Psychological Effects of Marijuana in Man." *Science* 162 (1968): 1234 ff.

Chapter 6

Hallucinogens: LSD and Others

As indicated in Chapter 1, there are many chemical substances that have the power to influence the way a person thinks, feels, and perceives the world. Cortico-steroid drugs, for example, which are commonly used in the diagnosis and treatment of adrenal disorders, severe allergies, and skin diseases are capable of producing symptoms that are not dissimilar to those seen in mental illness. These symptoms may include mood alterations, nervousness, depression, and overexcitement. In such cases, the psychological changes induced by the drug are viewed as unfortunate secondary, or side, effects, and use of the drug may be discontinued by the physician. In contrast, there are a number of other drugs which produce these same psychological changes as their *primary* action, and some people seek out these drugs precisely for their effects. Among the drugs that fall into this category are d-lysergic acid diethylamide (LSD), mescaline, peyote, psilocybin, dimethyl-tryptamine (DMT), diethyltryptamine (DET), and 2,5 dimethoxy-4-methylamphetamine (DOM) as well as others. These drugs are referred to collectively as psychedelics, hallucinogens, psychotomimetics, or psychotogenics. These terms are briefly defined as follows:

1. The word *hallucinogen* refers to the ability of certain drugs to produce hallucinations or sensory experiences which do not correspond to external reality. An auditory hallucination may involve hearing voices, whereas a visual one may involve seeing the world differently than it really is.
2. The word *psychotomimetic* refers to the ability of LSD and related substances to "mimic" the *psychoses,* which are severe mental illnesses characterized by loss of contact with reality, hallucinations, and delusions (false beliefs held regardless of reality). This term is not entirely accurate in describing the effects of these drugs.
3. The word *psychedelic* refers to the so-called mind-expanding qualities of LSD and related substances. By "mind-expanding" is meant the ability to have a wider range of experiences while under the influence of these drugs than would otherwise be possible.
4. The word *psychotogenic* refers to the production of psychotic-like states.

The common characteristic of these drugs is that they can all produce feelings of unreality and loss of identity, as well as delusions, hallucinations, and extreme changes in mood.

Use of Hallucinogens

The use of drugs to induce hallucinations and other unusual experiences is not a new phenomenon. In fact, there is evidence to suggest that such drugs were probably in use as many as 5,000 years ago. In many parts of the world, hallucinogenic substances have long been used as part of religious or other ceremonies, and are still being used for such purposes today. For example, mescaline or peyote cactus was used centuries ago by the Aztec Indians in Mexico. And even today, peyote plays an important part of the religious ceremonies of certain North American Indian tribes, who use it in much the same way that the Christian religion uses bread and wine. In fact, until recently, peyote was still being sold through the mail. Another example is the use of psilocybin and psilocin, which are derived from the ''magic mushrooms'' of Central America and Mexico. The use of these mushrooms in religious rites probably dates back several thousand years, and is still a common practice today. One should not get the impression, however, that the use of hallucinogenic agents can only be found in the history of North and Central America. A hallucinogenic substance is found in the *Amanita muscaria* mushroom, which grows in Northern Europe and Russia. This mushroom, also known as *fly agaric,* contains two psychotomimetic agents, muscimol and ibotenic acid, both of which produce effects that are similar to those of LSD. It is now believed that this mushroom was used by the ancient Norse tribes before going into battle. It was taken by the warriors to bring about a state of intense rage. Our modern word ''berserk'' comes from the name of the ingredient found in this mushroom. Even today, the use of this hallucinogen continues among the tribes of Siberia.

LSD

Perhaps the best known of all the hallucinogenic drugs is d-lysergic acid diethylamide (LSD). Unlike mescaline, psilocybin, and muscimole, all of which are found in naturally occurring substances and have long histories of use, LSD is a relatively new drug, one that was discovered only a few decades ago. In 1943, a Swiss chemist named Albert Hofmann was conducting a series of experiments on LSD in his laboratory (at that time the drug had only been in existence about five years). During the course of his experimentation, Hofmann had an unusual experience, which he described as follows:

> Last Friday, April 16, 1943, I was forced to stop my work in the laboratory in the middle of the afternoon and to go home, as I was seized by a peculiar restlessness

> associated with a sensation of mild dizziness. Having reached home, I lay down and sank in a kind of drunkenness which was not unpleasant and which was characterized by extreme activity of imagination. As I lay in a dazed condition with my eyes closed (I experienced daylight as disagreeably bright) there surged upon me an uninterrupted stream of fantastic images of extraordinary plasticity and vividness and accompanied by an intense, kaleidoscope-like play of colors. This condition gradually passed off after about two hours.[1]

Because of Hofmann's belief that this strange experience was somehow related to the LSD, he deliberately took the drug again several days later. Taking what he thought to be a small dose, but what we now know to be a large one, he had an even more spectacular experience.

> As far as I remember, the following were the most outstanding symptoms: vertigo, visual disturbances; the faces of those around me appeared as grotesque, colored masks; marked motor unrest, alternating with paresis; an intermittent heavy feeling in the head, limbs, and the entire body, as if they were filled with metal; cramps in the legs, coldness and loss of feeling in the hands; a metallic taste on the tongue; dry, constricted sensation in the throat; feeling of choking; confusion alternating between clear recognition of my condition, in which state I sometimes observed, in the manner of an independent, neutral observer, that I shouted half insanely or babbled incoherent words. Occasionally I felt as if I were out of my body.[2]

Because the unusual experiences LSD caused were believed by some to be mimicking a psychosis (hence the term psychotomimetic), it was thought that the chemical could be used to study and understand psychoses such as schizophrenia. In addition, many persons thought that LSD (as well as other psychotomimetic drugs) might eventually be useful in the treatment of these mental disorders. (The usefulness of LSD for these purposes will be discussed later in this chapter.)

Effects of LSD

LSD seems to exert its effects upon certain specific areas of the brain and brain stem. It is almost always taken orally and generally produces its effects within thirty minutes to one hour after administration. It is a colorless, odorless, and tasteless substance, and only minute amounts (measured in micrograms or one one-thousandths of a milligram) are required to produce powerful psychological effects. Generally, LSD is added to a sugar cube or cracker to facilitate handling, and occasionally it may even be placed on a small piece of absorbent towel or cardboard. It is also available in capsule, tablet, or powder form. As with other illicit drugs, the user rarely knows exactly how much of the desired drug is actually present in the substance purchased. The effects of a single dose may last up to twelve hours.

Within one hour after LSD is administered, symptoms of stimulation of the sympathetic division of the autonomic nervous system become noticeable. These include an increased heart rate, increased blood pressure, and dilation of the pupils of the eyes. Trembling may also be present, as well as some lack of coordination.

The mechanism by which LSD produces its effects may involve two factors: (1) disruption of the serotonin balance of the brain (serotonin is a chemical transmitter of information between cells in the brain, and is necessary for proper brain functioning); and (2) lowering of the thresholds for stimulation of the nerve pathways which bring information into the brain, thus increasing the volume of signals coming into the brain. This effect may account in part for the vivid sensations experienced by LSD users while intoxicated.

Pattern of Use

The users of LSD are typically individuals who have already been exposed to marijuana. The most common pattern of use is to take the drug at intervals of a few weeks or months. As may be expected from what we already know about marijuana users, LSD users generally tend to be young, as well as better educated and more economically secure than are users of heroin and abusers of alcohol. They also tend to be people who are associated with subcultures or groups that value experiences of a religious or mystical nature, or who wish, for personal reasons, to experience different states of consciousness. Thus, a high proportion of LSD users may be found among college students, artists, or other individuals who are consciously seeking new forms of experience and awareness. Of course, among LSD users are those individuals who see the use of the drug as a symbol of their association with the counterculture. Another group of users consists of those persons who are using it to find some form of relief from their own problems, and think that in some magical fashion LSD may help them.

Dangers of Use

Like heroin, the use of LSD on a regular basis may result in the development of physiological tolerance. Naturally, when this occurs, increasingly larger doses of the drug are needed to achieve the desired effects. Unlike heroin, however, the symptoms of physiological withdrawal do not appear upon discontinuation of LSD. Thus, physical dependence on the drug does not occur. Although tolerance to LSD may develop quite rapidly, it also disappears rapidly—either process may take no more than a week.

LSD is not considered to be a lethal substance, and there are no known cases of death resulting from an overdose of the drug. However, LSD is by no means a harmless substance, and its use may carry substantial risks for the individual (as well as to an unborn child, if the user should happen to be pregnant). Perhaps the greatest amount of risk is to those individuals who have significant psychological problems at the time that they use LSD. Included in this group are persons who have severe neurotic, psychotic, hysterical, psychopathic, or depressive tendencies. Under the influence of LSD, such persons may become overtly psychotic, a condition which could lead them to act out their aggressive impulses. They can become dangerous to others or perhaps even attempt suicide. Even among relatively normal individuals, LSD use involves a certain amount of risk. ''Bad trips,'' characterized by severe panic reactions and occasionally by such physical symptoms as lack of coordination, blurred speech, difficulty in walking, disorientation, paranoid delusions, visual hallucinations, severe anxiety, and even convulsions, may occur. This type of reaction lasts up to twenty-four hours and is especially likely to occur when LSD is taken in conjunction with methamphetamine, which is not a uncommon practice.[3] The symptom that is most commonly seen, however, is a person who experiences panic during an LSD experience and may exhibit highly self-destructive behavior, such as rushing from a house to ''escape,'' or may have the terrifying feeling of being completely out of touch with reality.

Although no one can predict the exact reaction that an LSD user will experience, several factors are commonly known to affect the nature of the ''trip'':

1. The user's expectations of the drug's effects.
2. The amount of experience the user has had with LSD and other hallucinogens.
3. Concurrent or recent use of other drugs.
4. The context in which the drug is used—that is, whether it is used among friends in a familiar environment, or in a strange place where disapproving or unknown persons are present.

Treatment for a ''bad trip'' usually involves the administration of tranquilizers, medication to reduce anxiety and induce sleep, and personal support and reassurance by others.

There is also some evidence suggesting that regular use of high doses of LSD may result in irreversible chromosomal damage and permanent genetic effects. Birth defects as well as disorders of pregnancy, including spontaneous miscarriage, have been known to occur. The extent and exact nature of these effects have not yet been conclusively determined.[4]

One of the most widely reported adverse effects of LSD use is the phenomenon known as the ''flashback.'' This refers to the sudden involuntary and unexpected recurrence of the drug-induced experience, which may have taken place at some time in the past. Flashbacks may occur weeks or even months after LSD was originally used; sometimes they occur as much as a year later. The flashback may be a very frightening experience since it sometimes involves strong feelings of anxiety, accompanied by disturbances of all the senses, including vision, hearing, taste, smell, and so forth. During a flashback, which may occur following the use of any hallucinogen, the individual may have the distinct impression that he or she is under the influence of LSD once again. Flashbacks are particularly harmful to unstable individuals in whom the unexpected experience could trigger suicidal or psychotic behavior.

It has also been suggested that LSD may cause permanent brain damage, and that prolonged use may result in alterations of the user's personality, thus causing permanent changes in the manner of thinking and behaving. But none of these theories has been conclusively proven to date.

Peyote (or Mescaline)

Earlier in this chapter, it was noted that the use of the peyote cactus is still a common practice among Indians in the southwestern United States. The use of this substance, first described by the Spanish, has been practiced for many centuries, and apparently has its origins in the ancient Aztec tribes of Mexico. During the past century its use has spread to many Indian tribes in Mexico, as well as to tribes in this country and some in Canada. Today peyote is used (legally) in the rituals of the Native American Church and in the religious ceremonies of the Mescalero Indians in Mexico.

The peyote cactus is indigenous to the central and northern Mexican desert. The local tribes make ceremonial trips to collect the cactus; tribes that are located farther from the source can purchase the substance through the mail.

Although peyote contains more than fifteen active ingredients, the one that is largely responsible for producing hallucinations is *mescaline*. Mescaline in its pure form is used less often than is peyote, which is consumed in the form of "mescal buttons." These small, hard discs are sliced off from the crown of the peyote cactus and then dried. Once in this form, they are moistened by the saliva in the mouth and then swallowed. Mescaline in its pure form produces a different effect than peyote since peyote contains mescaline plus other hallucinogens.

Peyote intoxication, which develops gradually once the drug has been ingested, is characterized by visual, auditory, and tactile hallucinations. The visual hallucinations may take the form of "visions" in which the user sees extremely beautiful colors and bright lights. Many users report having been able to "see" auditory stimuli (or sounds) while intoxicated, and some say that these sounds can be seen in color. This phenomenon of cross-modality perception is called *synesthesia*. Accompanying these psychological symptoms are several unpleasant physical symptoms, including nausea, increased heart rate, headaches, tremors, and profuse perspiration. Excitation is also present, as well as a feeling of anxiety. The entire episode lasts about twelve hours, and is generally followed by a period of deep sleep.

Many drug users claim that the effects of peyote and mescaline are similar to those of LSD, but most of these express a preference for the latter. In addition, because LSD is usually easier to obtain, its use is more common than that of peyote and and mescaline.

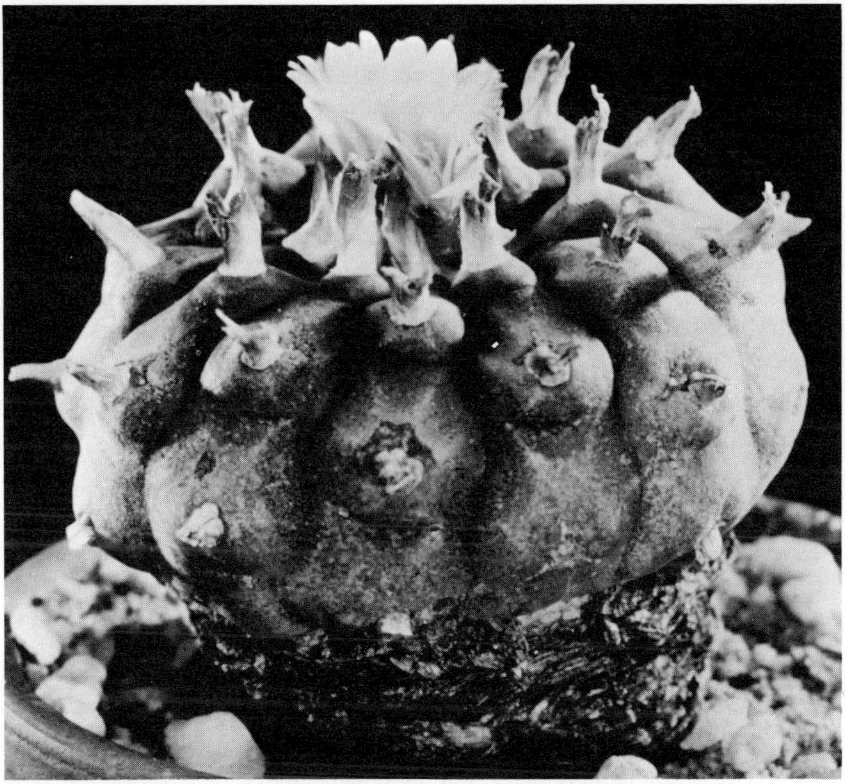

SOURCE: Drug Enforcement Administration, U.S. Department of Justice
Figure 6. This photograph of the peyote cactus clearly shows a flower in bloom on the body of the plant, which is light green in color, as well as the characteristic tufts of white hairs. The dried stem of this plant contains mescaline, which produces strong visual hallucinations, characterized by their intense and beautiful color.

Like LSD, mescaline and peyote do not produce physical dependence, but when these drugs are taken on a regular basis (which is rarely the case), the development of tolerance can result.

DOM (STP)

DOM is the biochemical abbreviation for a powerful hallucinogen which first appeared in 1967. The chemical structure of this substance resembles that of both mescaline *and* amphetamine, and thus belongs to a group of psychoactive substances called the psychotomimetic amphetamines. The effects of DOM are so potent, in fact, that it was given the nickname ''STP'' by users (STP is a well-known gasoline additive). The implication is that the drug somehow improves brain performance. Another interpretation of the meaning of these initials is "Serenity, Tranquility, and Peace."

Taken orally in capsule or tablet form, the effects produced by DOM are similar to those described for LSD and mescaline—with the addition of marked elation and excitement. There is also the occasional feeling of being overwhelmed by stimuli from the environment, as well as an inability to distinguish a good "trip" from a bad one. Although it was originally believed that the effects of DOM could last up to three days, it is now known that the actual duration of effect is about seven to nine hours. There are many reports, however, of the effects having lasted as long as twenty-four hours. Many adverse reactions are associated with this drug and as a consequence its usage has decreased significantly since it was first introduced several years ago.

Psilocybin and Psilocin

Psilocybin and psilocin are psychoactive substances derived from a group of mushrooms known as *Psilocybe mexicana*. These mushrooms have long been used in the religious ceremonies of certain Mexican Indian tribes, who refer to them as "God's flesh." Psilocybin and psilocin, when taken orally in liquid or powdered form, rapidly produces physical and psychological effects that are similar to those of LSD and mescaline. However, psilocybin has a much more calming effect than LSD and mescaline, which, as we have seen, also produce excitement. The effects of psilocybin and psilocin reach a peak between one and two hours after administration, and last for a total of four to six hours. Thus, the onset of action is more rapid, but the effects have a shorter duration. The intensity of the psilocybin experience is largely determined by the dose level. Small doses may produce a mild, pleasant experience, whereas large doses may involve strong visual and other hallucinatory experiences, which could be quite unpleasant.

Minor Hallucinogens

In addition to the more widely used hallucinogens, such as LSD, mescaline, DOM, and psilocybin, there are a number of less widely known (and less frequently used) substances. These include DMT, harmine, bufotenine, and fly agaric, all of which are naturally occurring substances. These drugs tend to be used as intoxicants rather than as hallucinogens.

Bufotenine

This substance, which is called yopo by South American Indians, has been used in Haiti and in certain parts of South America as a narcotic snuff. It is found in the secretions of the skin glands of toads as well as in certain plants, the seeds of which are crushed to make the snuff. Bufotenine produces a state of

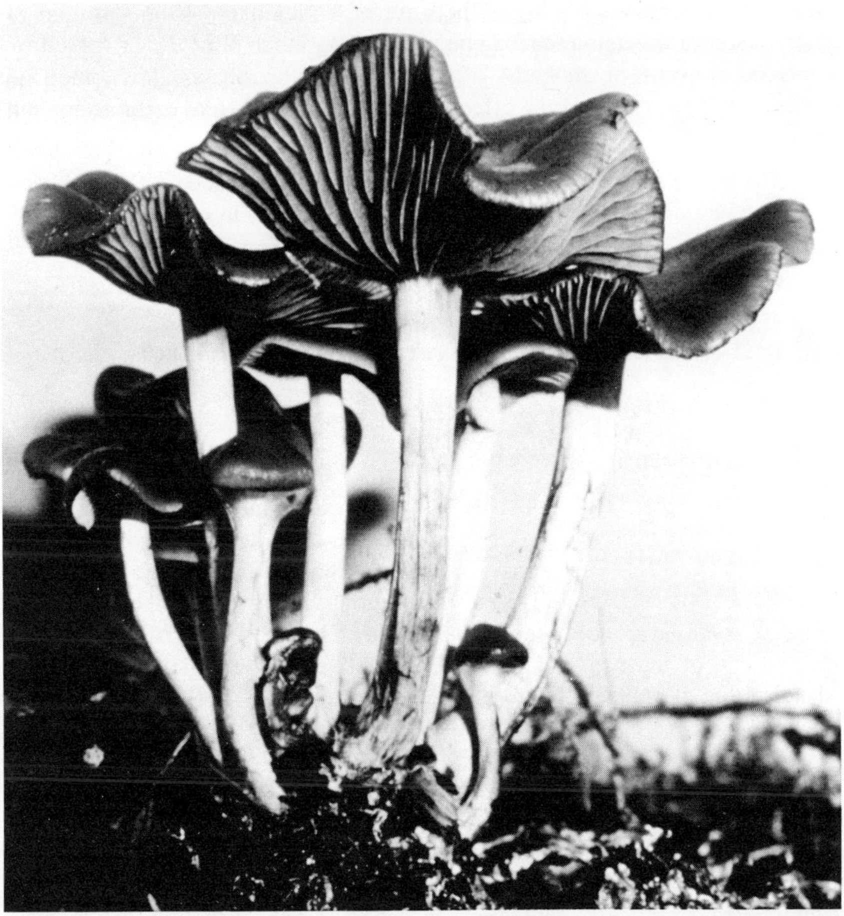

SOURCE: Drug Enforcement Administration, U.S. Department of Justice
Figure 7. Psilocybe mushrooms. These mushrooms, upon ingestion, cause intense hallucinations as well as disturbances of time and space similar to those caused by LSD.

intoxication that is similar to that produced by LSD and psilocybin, although with bufotenine, there are less complex visual disturbances as well as strong physical side effects, including reddening and swelling of the face, difficulty in walking, and some degree of paralysis. The physical effects appear first, followed by excitement, and ending in drugged sleep.

DMT (Dimethyltryptamine)

This substance represents an important component of such South American snuffs as bufotenine. It is more widely used outside the United States but does occasionally turn up in this country. It is often referred to as the "businessman's

LSD'' or ''businessman's high'' because of its relatively short duration of action, a sort of diversion that can be used during lunch hour. DMT can either be inhaled as a snuff or smoked—often it is mixed with tobacco. It is somewhat similar to LSD in terms of the effects it produces, but differs in the following important ways.

1. The effects of DMT appear much more rapidly than do those of LSD, but they also subside much more rapidly, in perhaps only thirty to sixty minutes.
2. Physical and psychological symptoms appear simultaneously.
3. DMT alters only visual perceptions—it does not affect auditory or tactile sensations.
4. DMT causes lack of coordination and spasticity, an effect not characteristic of LSD.

Ololiuqui (Morning Glory)

Another hallucinogenic substance used by South American Indians is found in the seeds of the morning glory plant. When eaten, the seeds of this plant produce psychoactive effects that are similar to those of LSD; they also produce such physical side effects as nausea and vomiting, intense headache, and drowsiness. The similarities between ololiuqui and LSD are not surprising, considering that one of the active ingredients in ololiuqui is lysergic acid amide, a substance that is chemically closely related to LSD.

Fly Agaric

As mentioned earlier in the chapter, the use of fly agaric *(Amanita muscaria)* first originated in Europe many centuries ago. This substance, which is found in certain mushrooms, derives its name from its use as a fly poison. When used for hallucinogenic purposes, however, fly agaric is either swallowed whole or mixed with milk or water. The psychotomimetic state produced by this substance is not as intense as that produced by LSD or psilocybin. According to one description of the effects of *Amanita muscaria,*

> an hour after the ingestion of the mushrooms, twitching and trembling of the limbs is noticeable with the onset of a period of good humor and light euphoria, characterized by macroscopia, visions of the supernatural, and illusions of grandeur. Religious overtones—such as an urge to confess sins—frequently occur. Occasionally, the partaker becomes violent, dashing madly about until, exhausted, he drops into a deep sleep.[5]

The effects of fly agaric vary from individual to individual.

There are two other points to be made about fly agaric. First, this mushroom may be the cause in some cases that are diagnosed as mushroom poisoning. The person may not be suffering from mushroom poisoning at all. Second, fly agaric is excreted in the urine without being chemically changed. Thus, a not uncommon practice among users of this drug is to "recycle" the urine of a person who is intoxicated.

Nutmeg and Mace

Nutmeg and mace are two common household spices whose psychedelic properties have been discovered only recently. When brewed into a tea or otherwise ingested in *large* amounts, both nutmeg and mace can produce strong visual hallucinations and other disturbances of perception, as well as a general feeling of euphoria. These effects are probably due to the fact that both spices contain myristicin and elemicin, two substances that are closely related to mescaline. The use of nutmeg and mace as psychedelic agents produces strong side effects, including vomiting, nausea, and tremors.

Because of their ready availability in the kitchens of correctional facilities, the use of nutmeg and mace to obtain a "high" has been a frequent occurrence in such institutions.

MDA

MDA (3,4-methylenedioxyamphetamine) is a psychotomimetic drug that is closely related to DOM (STP). Like DOM, it has the characteristics of both mescaline and amphetamine. MDA—or the "love-drug," as it is called on the street—is usually taken orally in capsule, tablet, or liquid form although it may also be injected or sniffed ("snorted"). The effects of MDA, which become noticeable about one hour after taking the drug and last for approximately eight hours, typically include mild euphoria, a desire to interact positively with others, and a heightened sense of emotional and physical awareness. MDA does not produce the visual and auditory hallucinations characteristic of LSD intoxication. Although it is known that MDA is a stimulant, little is known about its effects on the body or its side effects. It has been suggested that MDA might be useful as an adjunct in psychotherapy.

PCP (Phencyclidine)

Phencyclidine was originally used as a surgical anesthetic (under the trade name Sernyl), but when it was found to have strong side effects, which included excitation, disturbances of vision, and delirium, its medical use was discontinued. The drug was used illegitimately for a while and was marketed on the street under the name PCP ("peace pill"). PCP was not only sold as a hallucinogen in its own right but was a frequent substitute for mescaline, cocaine, and THC (the active ingredient in marijuana). PCP has also appeared on the street under the pseudonyms "hog" and "angel dust." The latter refers to the use of PCP by sprinkling it over marijuana or tobacco, which is then smoked. It is also ingested orally, usually in capsules. PCP produces unpleasant effects, including loss of identity (depersonalization), visual and auditory hallucinations, loneliness, isolation, and depression. Psychotic episodes or attempted suicides are not uncommon in PCP users. Because of these serious psychological and physical side effects, and the variable effects obtained at different dose levels, deliberate use of PCP on the street has dropped off. However, PCP continues to be substituted for other drugs, such as THC, LSD, and mescaline.

Are Psychedelic Drugs Useful in Treating Mental Illness?

During early studies of the effects of LSD on human beings, investigators made an interesting observation. They discovered that some of their subjects, while under the influence of the drug, were able to vividly remember significant, and sometimes traumatic, events from their past—events that had previously been repressed. In some cases, the subjects were even able to relive the emotional experiences of these events. The discovery of this phenomenon, which in psychotherapy is called abreaction, led some therapists to consider the possibility of using LSD in the treatment of emotional disorders, and many became convinced that it might be highly useful for this purpose.[6]

Some reports suggested that in addition to allowing the patient to uncover and relive previously repressed emotional experiences, LSD might also be useful in psychotherapy in a number of other ways.

1. Because LSD reduces feelings of defensiveness, it might effectively increase the patient's confidence in the therapist.
2. Under the influence of LSD the patient becomes more objective, in part because there is a feeling of being more detached from one's problems.
3. LSD increases the range of emotional expressiveness on the part of the patient, and increases the ability to communicate with the therapist.
4. LSD allows the patient to achieve a higher level of personality integration and self-acceptance, as well as basic changes in values and beliefs.

If the above claims for LSD could be found to be valid, then the drug would certainly prove to be an invaluable tool in the treatment of psychiatric disorders. But the fact is that studies conducted thus far to test the therapeutic usefulness of LSD have not consistently supported these claims. For instance, one study found that when LSD was used in the treatment of a group of alcoholics with a low likelihood of recovery, some 49 percent showed much improvement and another 26 percent showed some improvement.[7] Another study, which also focused on the usefulness of LSD in the treatment of alcoholics, found it to be no more effective than other forms of treatment; in fact, the patients seemed to improve regardless of the type of treatment they received. Thus, LSD was shown to have no special usefulness in the treatment of alcoholics.[8] It should be remembered that while there are many advocates of the use of LSD in therapy,[9] there are just as many who feel it is not useful for this purpose and even a few who believe that LSD therapy may be detrimental to some individuals.[10] The fact that it is often difficult to predict how a person will react to LSD poses a major problem for its use in therapy. Obviously, further research is needed in this area in order to determine whether LSD actually possesses the positive therapeutic effects that have been attributed to it.

Do Hallucinogens Enhance Creativity?

It is popularly believed among members of the drug subculture that LSD and other hallucinogens stimulate creativity. Although it is true that under the influence of these substances an individual may produce very original, unusual, and perhaps creative works of art, or may think of new and novel ways of solving problems, it is difficult to determine exactly what role the hallucinogen itself plays in this heightened creativity. It may be that these drugs stimulate the creative process by allowing new and novel associations, or more likely by removing blocks that stand in the way of creativity, such as self-criticism, anxiety, fear of failure, and other factors that normally inhibit creative expression. It is also possible that, for a while at least, these drugs actually increase the rate at which new ideas are produced. But they probably also increase the rate at which poor ideas are produced. Thus, one could conclude that with a greater number of ideas being produced, a useful one might prove to be present among them.

Although drugs may be useful in enhancing creativity, there are many other means of achieving the same end. F. Leavitt, in the following excerpt from an excellent chapter on the role of drugs in creativity, makes some interesting observations on this issue:

> Brainstorming and its variants, meditation, biofeedback conditioning, courses in painting and creative writing . . . all of these have the virtue of being legal and probably safe, and some are of proven effectiveness. Results are not immediate, which is one of the attractions of the claims for hallucinogens. A more important difference between drugs and alternatives to them is that the latter are concerned primarily with improving technique; hallucinogens on the other hand, if they have any value, are effective by virtue of providing new perspectives which provide challenges to basic assumptions about the nature and function of art.[11]

Notes

1. A. Hofmann, "Psychotomimetic Agents," in A. Burger, ed., *Drugs Affecting the Central Nervous System,* Vol. 2 (New York: Dekker, 1968), pp. 184 ff.
2. Ibid.
3. M. Reidenberg and D. Lowenthal, "Adverse Nondrug Reactions," *New England Journal of Medicine* 279 (1968): pp. 678–679.

4. R. M. Julian, *A Primer of Drug Action* (San Francisco: Freeman, 1975), pp. 76–77.

5. R. E. Schultes, "Hallucinogens of Plant Origin," *Science* 163 (1969): p. 246.

6. J. C. Coleman, *Abnormal Psychology and Modern Life,* 3rd ed. (Glenview, Ill.: Scott, Foresman, 1964), p. 584.

7. J. R. MacLean et al., "The Use of LSD-25 in the Treatment of Alcoholism and Other Psychiatric Problems," *Quarterly Journal of Studies on Alcohol* 22 (1961): pp. 34–45.

8. G. Johnson, "LSD in the Treatment of Alcoholism," *American Journal of Psychiatry* 126 (1969): pp. 481–487.

9. A. Hoffer and H. Osmond, *The Hallucinogens* (New York: Academic Press, 1967).

10. S. Cohen, "Lysergic Acid Diethylamide: Side Effects and Complications," *Journal of Nervous and Mental Diseases* 130 (1960): pp. 30–40.

11. F. Leavitt, *Drugs and Behavior* (Philadelphia: Saunders, 1974), p. 305.

Selected Bibliography

Buckman, J. "Social and Medical Aspects of Illicit Use of LSD." *International Journal of Social Psychiatry* 17 (1971): 163–176.

Hofmann, F. G. *A Handbook on Drug and Alcohol Abuse.* New York: Oxford, 1975.

Horowitz, M. J. "Flashbacks: Recurrent Intrusive Images After the Use of LSD." *American Journal of Psychiatry* 126 (1969): 565–569.

Jaffe, J. H. "Drug Addiction and Drug Abuse." In Goodman, L. S., and Gilman, A., eds. *The Pharmacological Basis of Therapeutics,* 4th ed. New York: Macmillan, 1970.

Julien, R. M. *A Primer of Drug Action.* San Francisco: Freeman, 1975.

Longo, V. G. *Neuropharmacology and Behavior.* San Francisco: Freeman, 1975.

McGothin, W. H.; Sparkes, R. S.; and Arnold, D. O. "Effect of LSD on Human Pregnancy." *Journal of the American Medical Association* 212 (1970): 1483 ff.

National Clearinghouse for Drug Abuse Information. *DOM (STP),* 1973. Report Series 17, No. 1, 1973.

Ray, O. S. *Drugs, Society, and Human Behavior.* St. Louis: Mosby, 1972.

Schultes, R. E. "Hallucinogens of Plant Origin." *Science* 163 (1969): 245–254.

Smart, R. G., and Bateman, K. "Unfavorable Reactions to LSD: A Review and Analysis of the Available Case Reports." *Canadian Medical Association Journal* 97 (1967): 1214 ff.

Smart, R. G., and Bateman, K. "The Chromosomal and Teratogenic Effects of Lysergic Acid Diethylamide: A Review of the Current Literature." *Canadian Medical Association Journal* 99 (1968): 805 ff.

Zegans, L. S.; Pollard, J. C.; and Brown, D. "The Effects of LSD-25 on Creativity and Tolerance to Regression." *Archives of General Psychiatry* 16 (1967): 748 ff.

Chapter 7

Stimulants: Amphetamines and Cocaine

This chapter will survey the most commonly abused stimulants, many of which have at one time or another had useful medical applications. For example, the amphetamines have been used to dilate the bronchial tubes in the lungs in cases of asthma (a common example is the inhaler marketed under the well-known name Benzedrine), and to treat such diverse disorders as narcolepsy,* obesity, Parkinson's disease, petit mal epilepsy, and depression. The amphetamines have also been used as an antidote to overdoses of depressants, and to maintain alertness under conditions of fatigue—for example, amphetamine tablets have been used by soldiers and sailors during wartime to help them maintain a high level of alertness.

Cocaine was the first local anesthetic ever used and today it is still being used for this purpose in preparations for the nose, throat, and eye. The barbiturates and tranquilizers also have many beneficial uses. All of these drugs, however, have a common property which results in their relatively widespread abuse. This property is simply their ability to alter a person's level of activity or arousal. The depressants *reduce* levels of activity whereas the stimulants *increase* them.

Amphetamines: Use and Abuse

Amphetamine is a powerful stimulant of central nervous system (CNS) activity. Among the direct effects produced by initial oral doses of 10 to 30 mg of this drug are the following:

1. Increased levels of wakefulness and alertness.
2. Decreased feelings of fatigue and increase in energy, mood elevation, and feelings of confidence.

*A form of epilepsy characterized by uncontrollable attacks of sleeping, which may occur many times a day.

3. Decreased reaction time.
4. Increased ability to concentrate.
5. Decreased appetite.
6. Increased threshold for pain perception.

All of the above are highly desirable effects for individuals in certain types of situations—for instance, when high levels of vigilance and alertness must be maintained in a combat situation. Other groups of individuals besides military personnel have used amphetamines to take advantage of some of these effects. Among these are truck drivers on long trips, students seeking to stay awake in order to study for exams, athletes seeking to enhance their performances, and obese persons seeking to lose weight. The usefulness of amphetamines to these individuals may be less than expected, however, and this issue will be touched upon below.

Side Effects

Some side effects may accompany the above primary effects. These can include:

1. Increased activity and restlessness
2. Increased irritability
3. Increased sexual drive
4. Dilated pupils
5. Dry mouth
6. Heart palpitations
7. Increased speed and decreased clarity of speech
8. Muscle tremors
9. Headaches and nausea
10. Decreased coordination
11. Grinding of the teeth

The extent to which these symptoms appear in any given individual will of course depend upon such factors as the size of the dose administered, the personality of the user, and the individual's psychological state at the time the dose is administered.

After the drug has begun to wear off, there is frequently a "washed out" feeling, often accompanied by psychological depression and sleep. Surprisingly, the user experiences little or no "hangover" upon awakening from this drug-induced sleep.

Medical Uses

The amphetamines, which were first synthesized in the late nineteenth century, were not found to have medical uses until the late 1920s. The drug was first used in the treatment of asthma and related respiratory problems and was marketed for this purpose in an inhaler under the trade name Benzedrine. Since 1949, however, the amphetamine content in Benzedrine inhalers has been replaced with other, less potent substances. This change was made because of the extent to which these inhalers were being abused.

Amphetamine in its various chemical forms (amphetamine sulfate, dextroamphetamine sulfate and phosphate) is usually a white powder and is available in capsule, tablet, and liquid forms. Dexedrine is the trade name for dextroamphetamine sulfate. Methamphetamine is closely related chemically to the other amphetamines but has stronger CNS effects and fewer physical effects. Methamphetamine is marketed under the trade names Methedrine, Desoxyn, and Syndrox, to name a few. Today, the medical uses of amphetamine are limited to the treatment of three types of problems. These uses reflect the restrictions placed on these drugs by the Federal Drug Administration in 1970.

1. *Narcolepsy.* Amphetamine is thought to be useful in treating this rare disorder which takes the form of brief attacks of deep sleep.
2. *Hyperactivity in children.* Amphetamine has been found to be useful in treating hyperactivity, which is also referred to as minimal brain damage or minimal brain dysfunction (MBD). However, other drugs which are now available may be more useful. Why amphetamine, which is itself a stimulant, should be useful in treating problems of hyperactivity is not completely understood.
3. *Short-term treatment of obesity.* Amphetamine has been found to be an effective appetite depressant for periods of up to six weeks—that is, unless the dose is substantially increased. It does not, however, affect the basic cause of obesity—habitual overeating—which soon reappears once the drug has been discontinued. The dieter who uses amphetamines usually returns to the original weight level after a short time.

Nonmedical Uses

A high proportion of the legal amphetamines produced in this country each year cannot be accounted for in terms of prescriptions. In addition, the production of amphetamines in home "laboratories" is believed to be quite substantial. Thus, there is a considerable amount of amphetamine available for sale, often at relatively low prices. However, availability of the drug cannot by itself explain why it is so widely abused. Among the reasons suggested for this abuse are the fact that (1) amphetamines are well known to the public; (2) they are readily available; and (3) they are effective in meeting the perceived needs of users—for example, in maintaining high levels of activity in work, recreation, or sex, in temporarily relieving depression, and in gratifying needs for sensation and stimulation.

Pattern of Use

Generally, there are several different types of amphetamine users. These types can be categorized under three degrees of use.

Intermittent low-dose use. Intermittent low-dose use means use for purposes of avoiding onset of fatigue, maintaining wakefulness, decreasing boredom while carrying out repetitive tasks, and occasional use to get ''high.'' Amphetamines are usually obtained from friends; no particular age pattern is associated with this kind of abuse. The usual dose may be 5 to 20 mg taken orally. This type of use is typical of those who want short-term results such as students and truck drivers.

Sustained low-to-moderate-dose use. In cases of low-to-moderate use, amphetamines may be obtained legitimately (usually for weight-reducing purposes) and used three to four times daily as a means of attaining a state of euphoria and increased self-confidence. The individual who obtains Benzedrine from an inhaler would fall into this category. At first, the drug may be used daily or only on weekends. Psychological dependence may develop, as well as withdrawal symptoms. Because amphetamines cause sleeplessness, sedatives, or downers, are often used to induce sleep.

High-dose intravenous methamphetamine use. Intravenous use, described in greater detail below, is associated with the ''speed freak,'' or ''needle freak,'' the individual whose pattern of life is as strongly influenced by the use of amphetamines as is the heroin addict's by the use of opiates. This type of abuser, who may begin using oral amphetamines as an adolescent, eventually ''graduates'' to the point where he or she is injecting either methamphetamine, amphetamine, or both. When injected, these drugs produce an immediate feeling of euphoria and pleasure called the ''flash'' allegedly similar to the ''rush'' produced by heroin. This heavy use may be sustained for days at a time.

Long-term Effects

There are clearly dangers associated with the chronic use of amphetamines. This is particularly true during periods of intense high-dosage use (''runs'') which are followed by a period of exhaustion after termination of use of the drug (the ''crash''). These may include:

1. The danger of a psychotic state persisting after the run has ended.
2. The risk of suicide during a crash and its accompanying depression.

3. The intravenous method of taking the drug subjects the user to the same risks of infection as the heroin addict (see Chapter 4).
4. Chronic states of excitement and/or suspiciousness (paranoia) and general personality deterioration.
5. Impairment of memory and ability to concentrate.
6. The possibility of brain damage.
7. Significant weight loss and malnutrition as a result of starvation while a run is in progress.

The "Speed Freak"

As noted above, the intravenous use of amphetamines or methamphetamine is usually associated with a pattern of abuse which involves periodic sprees or runs, periods of intense use lasting anywhere from three days to one or more weeks. During this time doses equivalent to 100 to 3,000 mg of amphetamines may be taken every two or three hours (to appreciate the size of these dosages, recall that a dose of 5 to 10 mg is normally sufficient to produce the stimulant effects described earlier).

The effects of the flash or rush which the user usually experiences before removing the needle from the vein has been likened by some users to an intense sexual orgasm. Because the effects of the drug soon begin to wane, there is a frequent re-injection of amphetamines. While high, the user may be extremely expansive and euphoric, have feelings of omnipotence and confidence, and be unusually excitable and hyperactive. In some cases sexual desire may be increased, but in others it may either decrease or not be affected at all. When sexual activity is engaged in, orgasm may be delayed and the sexual experience made more intense.

In addition to the symptoms described above, the heavy amphetamine user may also have difficulty swallowing and urinating, heart palpitations, and increased blood pressure. But these effects are insignificant compared to the psychological effects of an amphetamine run.

Psychologically, the amphetamine run results in a general deterioration of the user's personality.

1. *Amphetamine psychosis.* Amphetamine psychosis is characterized by frightening hallucinations and visions, and the development of paranoid suspiciousness. Such suspiciousness may lead to feelings of persecution (paranoia), with friends being seen as police informers, and strangers as enemies. These incorrect beliefs as well as the general distortion of the cognitive processes may result in potential explosiveness, so that violence could occur.
2. *Compulsive behavior.* During the amphetamine run the user may engage in repetitive acts such as cleaning and polishing objects over and over, or straightening and restraightening the objects on a bureau. This behavior is accompanied by a loss of interest in the outside world.

3. *Tactile hallucinations.* The user may develop the sensation of bugs crawling over the skin. These "cocaine bugs," as they are called, may become so annoying that the user may be injured in attempting to kill or remove them with a knife or by picking at the skin.

Eventually, the run must end, due to a short supply of the drug, total physical exhaustion, a deliberate decision on the part of the user, or a fear of injections caused by drug-induced paranoia. The run is said to end in a crash. This consists of a deep sleep, perhaps lasting several days, followed by depression, anxiety, and general emotional discomfort, which may last for weeks. Often the crash is so intense that it leads either to thoughts of suicide or to the notion of beginning another run as a means of escape.

Amphetamine Addiction

Obviously, the way in which amphetamines are abused by the speed freak differs significantly from the pattern of abuse observed in the truck driver seeking to stay awake on a long trip or the housewife seeking to counteract boredom and lethargy. Since neither of these is likely to become a speed freak, it can be said that amphetamines do not create the level of physical dependency that the narcotics do. Therefore, amphetamine abuse should be considered in light of the purpose served by the drug. Viewed in this way, each of the three groups of users described above uses the drug to meet its own needs. The needs of the truck driver and the bored housewife are evident, but what are the needs of the speed freak? The individuals in this group are typically emotionally unstable, and often have histories of police contacts, homosexuality, or alcohol abuse. Such individuals are often sensation-seekers, persons who orient their lives around satisfying their needs quickly and obtaining as many highs as possible—needs that are more closely met by the amphetamines than by narcotics or alcohol. Psychological dependence develops as use continues, and tolerance leads to even larger doses being used. Thus, even though physical dependence may not be evident, the individual can become addicted to amphetamine as readily as others become addicted to heroin.

Cocaine

Cocaine, also known as "snow," "coke," or "the rich man's drug," was in regular use among South American Indians even before the Spanish arrived. The Indians did not know the drug in the white powder form we know today, but rather as leaves of the *Erythroxylon coca* shrub, which they chewed to extract the active ingredient. These leaves were valued so highly by the Indians that they constituted a form of currency, a practice which was continued by the Spanish, who paid their Indian workers with it. Not until the ninteenth century was the active ingredient of this plant isolated. Incidently, contrary to popular belief, this plant has nothing to do with the cocoa plant.

Cocaine has an extremely colorful history. Following are some of the more interesting historical facts associated with its use.

1. About 800 to 1,000 years ago, coca leaves were used as a local anesthetic in *trephining* operations (the boring of holes in the skull).
2. Dr. Sigmund Freud, the father of psychoanalysis, at one time advocated the use of cocaine in the treatment of a variety of ailments, including indigestion, asthma, and depression. He even used cocaine in an attempt to cure the opiate addiction of a friend, who then became addicted to cocaine.
3. Cocaine was the first anesthetic available for eye surgery, and was also used in dentistry until the development of a synthetic substance, procaine, replaced it. Incidently, procaine—or Novocain, as we are more likely to know it—has the anesthetic characteristics of cocaine without the stimulant effects.
4. Sherlock Holmes, the famous literary character, was, according to Dr. Watson, an abuser of cocaine, as perhaps his creator, Sir Arthur Conan Doyle, may have been.
5. The popular soft drink Coca-Cola originally had a small amount of cocaine as one of its ingredients. It no longer contains cocaine, but the trade name still is *Coca*-Cola.

After the passage of the Harrison Tax Act in 1914 (see Chapter 9), legitimate use of cocaine was limited to medical purposes. Cocaine had a following,

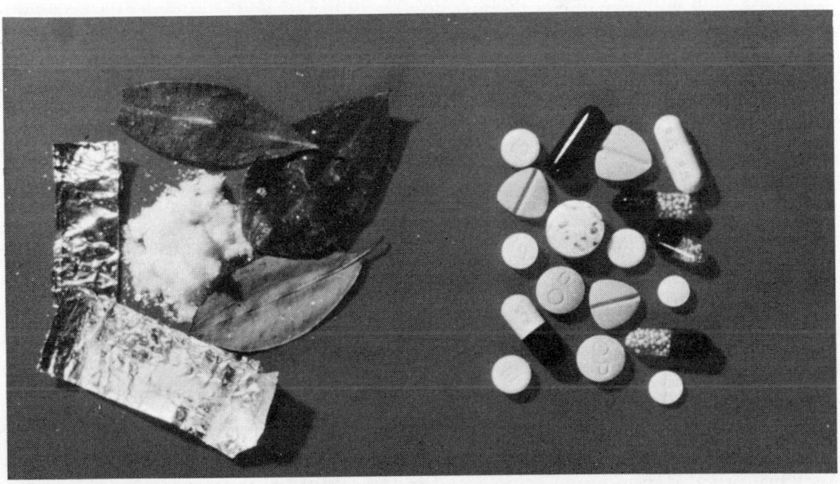

SOURCE: Drug Enforcement Administration, U.S. Department of Justice

Figure 8. Cocaine comes from the leaves of the coca bush. The leaves are sometimes chewed, particularly among the Indians in South America. The powdered form is most commonly used in the United States. Amphetamines tend to be found in a variety of shapes, colors, and sizes. Thus, the slang names such as "hearts," "peaches," "whites," "browns," and so forth.

however, and illegal traffic in it soon developed. Then, as today, cocaine was used only by a small number of individuals, its cost and scarcity being the limiting factors. Thus, cocaine is referred to as "the rich man's drug," and appropriately so since a "spoon" (1 g) of the drug, which is the usual unit of scale and which supplies five 200 mg "snorts," costs $50 to $200. However, as in the case of heroin, the spoon is likely to have been cut, or diluted, with other substances so that it is seldom more than 5 percent pure.

Effects of Cocaine

Cocaine abuse is in many ways similar to amphetamine abuse. This is not surprising when one learns that with a few exceptions, the effects of the two drugs are highly similar. The drug may either be inhaled or injected. According to Jaffe, "Cocaine addicts describe the euphoric effects of cocaine in terms that are almost indistinguishable from those used by amphetamine addicts."[1] In addition to the euphoric effects produced by cocaine, the following symptoms will be present:

1. There are the same subjective effects as those described above for amphetamine intoxication, including increased levels of wakefulness, alertness, and confidence, general elevation of mood, and decreased feelings of fatigue.
2. Sexuality is often stimulated, but for some individuals cocaine acts as an inhibitor of sexual motivation.
3. As with amphetamines, there is the possibility of inducing an active psychotic state with continued use during a run.
4. Cocaine has a shorter duration of action than amphetamine, and therefore doses are administered several times an hour.

Although many cocaine addicts claim that a better high can be obtained with cocaine, Jaffe disagrees.

> In short, while it is commonly assumed that the subjective effects of cocaine are more intense and its abuse potential more significant than those of the amphetamines, reliable evidence for this assumption is difficult to obtain . . .[2]

Side Effects

As may be expected, regular cocaine use produces many of the same side effects as those seen in amphetamine use. With regular use, tolerance and psychological dependence may develop. In addition, there are other dangers.

1. There is always a possibility of medical complications when any unsterile substance is injected.
2. Depression and apathy may follow the end of a run.
3. There is a risk of prolonged psychological effects, including the development of psychosis.

4. There is a chance that the nasal septum (the dividing wall between the two nasal cavities) may be perforated as a result of the prolonged constriction of blood vessels caused by regular sniffing of cocaine.
5. There is the risk of cocaine poisoning, which might result in breathing stoppage.
6. There is an occasional risk of almost immediate death due to interference with heart function.

Thus, there is really very little difference between cocaine and the amphetamines in terms of the effects produced. Considering cocaine's shorter duration of action and its higher cost, it is somewhat surprising that it should have such a favorable reputation among drug users.

Notes

1. J. H. Jaffe, "Drug Addiction and Drug Abuse," in L. S. Goodman and A. Gilman, eds., *The Pharmacological Basis of Therapeutics*, 4th ed. (New York: Macmillan, 1970), p. 293.
2. Ibid.

Selected Bibliography

Balster, R. L., and Schuster, C. R. "Fixed-interval Schedule of Cocaine Reinforcement: Effect of Dose and Infusion Duration." *Journal of the Experimental Analysis of Behavior* 20 (1973): 119–129.

Banarjee, U., and Lin, G. S. "On the Mechanism of Central Action of Amphetamine: The Role of Catecholamines." *Neuropharmacology* 12 (1973): 917–931.

Berger, H. J.; Brown, C. C.; and Krantz, J. C., Jr. "Fenfluramine Blockade of CNS Stimulant Effects of Amphetamines." *Journal of Pharmaceutical Sciences* 62 (1973): 788–791.

Borg, G.; Edstrom, C. G.; Linderholm, H.; and Marklund, G. "Changes in Physical Performance Induced by Amphetamine and Amobarbital." *Psychopharmacology* 26 (1972): 10–18.

Cappell, H.; Ginsberg, R.; and Webster, C. "Amphetamine and Conditioned 'Anxiety.'" *British Journal of Pharmacology* 45 (1972): 525–531.

Carey, R. J. "Disruption of Timing Behavior Following Amphetamine Withdrawal." *Physiological Pharmacology* 1 (1973): 9–12.

Clausen, J., and Fisher, S. "Effects of Amphetamine and Barbiturate on Body Experience." *Psychosomatic Medicine* 35 (1973): 390–405.

DeAlarcon, R. "An Epidemiological Evaluation of a Public Health Measure Aimed at Reducing the Availability of Methylamphetamine." *Psychological Medicine* 2 (1972): 293–300.

Domino, E. F.; Albers, J.; Potvin, A.; Repa, B.; and Tourtellotte, W. "Effects of d-Amphetamine on Quantitative Measures of Motor Performance." *Clinical Pharmacology and Therapeutics* 13 (1972): 251–257.

Ellinwood, E. H.; Sudilovsky, A.; and Grabowy, R. "Olfactory Forebrain Seizures Induced by Methamphetamine and Disulfiram." *Biological Psychiatry* 7 (1972): 89–99.

Evans, H. L.; Ghiselli, W. B.; and Patton, R. A. "Diurnal Rhythm in Behavioral Effects of Methamphetamine, p-Chloromethamphetamine, and Scopolamine." *Journal of Pharmacology and Experimental Therapeutics* 186 (1973): 10–17.

Gray, G. R.; Sheppard, C. W.; Inaba, D. S.; and Newmeyer, J. A. "An Old Girl: Flyin' Low, Dyin' Slow, Blinded by Snow: Cocaine in Perspective." *International Journal of the Addictions* 8 (1973): 1027–1042.

Grinspoon, L., and Hedblom, P. "Marijuana and Amphetamine: A Mirror Image." *Contemporary Drug Problems* 2 (1973): 665–682.

Groppetti, A. "Amphetamines and Cocaine on Amine Turnover." *Life Sciences* 13 (1973): lxii–lxiii.

Hall, C. D.; Blanton, D. E.; Scatliff, J. H.; and Morris, C. E. "Speed Kills: Fatality from the Self-administration of Methamphetamine Intravenously." *Southern Medical Journal* 66 (1973): 650–652.

Hendin, H. "Student Amphetamine Abuse." *Journal of Nervous and Mental Disease* 158 (1974): 256–267.

Hofmann, F. G. *A Handbook on Drug and Alcohol Abuse: The Biomedical Aspects*. New York: Oxford, 1975.

Milkman, H., and Frosch, W. A. "On the Preferential Abuse of Heroin and Amphetamine." *Journal of Nervous and Mental Disease* 156 (1973): 242–248.

Snyder, S. "Amphetamine Psychosis: A 'Model' Schizophrenia Mediated by Catecholamines." *American Journal of Psychiatry* 150 (1973): 61–67.

Watson, R. K.; Hartmann, E.; and Schildkraut, J. "Amphetamine Withdrawal. Affective State, Sleep Patterns, and MHPC Excretion." *American Journal of Psychiatry* 129 (1972): 263–269.

Part 2

TREATMENT, ENFORCEMENT AND PREVENTION, AND INVESTIGATION

Chapter 8

Treatment for Drug Abuse

One of the most serious challenges facing this country today is how to cope with the growing problem of drug abuse. In recent years, the number of Americans abusing dangerous drugs—particularly alcohol and narcotics—has reached massive proportions. It has been estimated that approximately five million people in this country have a severe drinking problem, and that some 5 to 10 percent of these eventually become chronic alcoholics. The number of narcotics addicts is equally staggering, with current estimates ranging from 800,000 to 1,000,000.[1]

These figures not only confirm the seriousness and scope of the problem, but they also point up the urgent need for effective methods of treating individuals suffering from drug addiction. Although there are many different forms of drug abuse, the two most prevalent—and dangerous—ones are alcoholism and heroin addiction. Thus, this chapter will be primarily concerned with the methods of treatment currently available to the alcoholic and the heroin addict. The first part of the chapter will examine the most commonly used methods of treating alcoholism; the remainder of the chapter will be devoted to the different types of treatment available to the heroin addict.

Treatment for the Alcoholic

Of the millions of individuals for whom the problem of alcoholism is a day-to-day reality, thousands each year seek treatment either for themselves or for an alcoholic who is a relative or a friend. There are many different types of alcoholics and, likewise, there are several different types of treatment from which the alcoholic can choose. Generally speaking, there is a rehabilitative approach that is appropriate for almost any type of alcohol abuser seeking treatment.

Of the many methods employed, the four that have proved most successful are psychotherapy, hospital outpatient treatment, conditioned reflex treatment, and fellowship and spiritual renewal. Naturally, within each of these categories there is some variation in technique, depending upon the practitioner(s) involved. Yet the commonalities are extensive enough to permit some general comments on each of the four types of treatment.

Psychotherapeutic Approaches

Psychotherapy, which is administered by a psychologist, psychiatrist, counselor, or psychiatric social worker, is geared toward helping the individual understand the motives underlying his or her alcoholic behavior so that the person can deliberately change it. In an atmosphere of acceptance and individual support, the alcoholic is encouraged to explore interpersonal and intrapsychic problems—some of which may be only indirectly related to drinking problems. The basic premise of the psychotherapeutic approach is that alcoholism represents a maladaptive behavior which can be corrected once the person gains a better self-understanding. The goal of psychotherapy, then, is to increase the alcoholic's self-awareness to the point where the alcoholic is motivated to make *initial* behavior changes on his or her own initiative.

Although psychotherapy is used extensively in the treatment of alcoholism and has proven to be quite effective, it nevertheless has considerable drawbacks. For one thing, it is often extremely expensive. Moreover, many alcoholics require a lengthy course of treatment, and even then its effectiveness is sometimes questionable.

Hospital Outpatient Treatment

Hospital outpatient treatment offers the alcoholic a number of services. In addition to medical attention, the alcoholic receives vitamin supplements as well as a number of other supports, including short-term counseling, group therapy, and a supply of antabuse, a drug which is incompatible with alcohol.

Conditioned Reflex Treatment

The conditioned reflex treatment involves the use of the drug antabuse. This drug is used because it induces vomiting in a person who drinks an alcoholic beverage after having taken it. The purpose of this form of treatment is that if the alcoholic experiences an adverse reaction (vomiting) every time a drink is taken, then the person will soon begin to associate alcohol with physical upset and will eventually withdraw from it.

Although the effects of antabuse last five to seven days after its administration, an obvious shortcoming of this approach is that its success depends on the cooperation of the alcoholic. Should the alcoholic decide to discontinue using the drug, after one week no further discomfort will be experienced. Moreover, some alcoholics drink in spite of antabuse's ill effects, and still others are only minimally affected by the drug.

Alcoholics Anonymous

Probably the most successful approach to treating alcoholism is that offered by Alcoholics Anonymous (A. A.). Alcoholics Anonymous is a nonprofessional organization that was founded by an ex-alcoholic and a medical doctor. By providing an environment of fellowship, spirituality, and mutual reinforcement, A. A. has helped literally thousands of alcoholics resolve their drinking problems. But the success of A. A. depends upon the alcoholic's willingness to make a sincere personal commitment to the objectives set forth by the organization.

One can get an idea of A. A.'s philosophical approach by reading the *Twelve Steps of Alcoholics Anonymous:*

1. We admitted we were powerless over alcohol—that our lives had become unmanageable.
2. Came to believe that a Power greater than ourselves could restore us to sanity.
3. Made a decision to turn our will and our lives over to the care of God *as we understood Him*.
4. Made a searching and fearless moral inventory of ourselves.
5. Admitted to God, to ourselves, and to another human being the exact nature of our wrongs.
6. Were entirely ready to have God remove all these defects of character.
7. Humbly asked Him to remove our shortcomings.
8. Made a list of all persons we had harmed, and became willing to make amends to them all.
9. Made direct amends to such people whenever possible, except when to do so would injure them or others.
10. Continued to take personal inventory, and when we were wrong, promptly admitted it.
11. Sought through prayer and meditation to improve our conscious contact with God, *as we understood Him,* praying only for knowledge of His will for us and the power to carry that out.
12. Having had a spiritual awakening as the result of these steps, we tried to carry this message to alcoholics and to practice these principles in all our affairs.*

Using this spiritual philosophy as a guideline, Alcoholics Anonymous attempts to help alcoholics rehabilitate themselves by encouraging them to reflect upon their behavior, and eventually to take corrective action so that they can become reintegrated into society.

Treatment for the Heroin Addict

The problem of how to control narcotics abuse—particularly heroin addiction—has long been a source of concern for criminal justice agencies. Two major approaches—punitive reaction and therapeutic intervention—have been tried in various forms, but all have had questionable success.

*Reprinted by permission of A. A. World Services, Inc.

The so-called legal, prohibitive, or punitive approaches were once the favored method of curbing drug abuse, but today these legal lock-up techniques are viewed as little more than stop-gap measures. (See Chapter 9.) The fact is that although imprisonment may prevent the drug abuser from taking drugs during the period of incarceration, there is no guarantee that the person won't begin abusing drugs again once he or she has been released.

Partly in reaction to the failure of the punitive approach, and partly because many believe that addiction should be viewed as an illness rather than as a crime, a number of new therapeutic approaches have been developed to help the narcotics abuser relinquish dependence on drugs. These techniques have been directed primarily toward the hard-drug abuser—that is, the heroin addict. Consequently, the remainder of this chapter will examine the methods used to treat the heroin abuser, since this segment of the drug population is of greatest concern to society.

Psychotherapeutic Approaches

Clarence Rowe, in *An Outline of Psychiatry,* sums up the reasons for the failure of traditional psychotherapy to rehabilitate drug abusers. "Ordinarily the prognosis is considered to be poor.[2] This should not be surprising since statistics have demonstrated that conventional psychotherapy is not always effective in treating even those for whom it was originally intended, much less nonneurotic addicts.

Moreover, many post-Freudian treatment theories developed for use with addicts are predicated on the notion that there is such a thing as an "addictive personality," but in fact it is questionable whether such a personality type exists at all. The fact is that although there are many intricate and sophisticated psychotherapeutic approaches to treating drug addicts, most of them simply do not work in practice.

One recent and fairly successful attempt to use a psychotherapeutic approach in treating drug addicts has been made by the proponents of so-called reality therapy. This method is purported to be somewhat different from conventional therapy.

> Reality therapy is designed to be a learning experience for the patient. It involves three steps. First, the patient must form an honest personal relationship with his therapist. . . . Next, the therapist must indicate to the patient that he understands, but does not condone, his irresponsible behavior. The patient's behavior is rejected, but he himself is accepted. Finally, the therapist teaches the patient better ways to fulfill his needs within the framework of reality (society as it exists).[3]

Of the incidences in which reality therapy has been used in the treatment of drug addicts, one therapist has reported a degree of success.[4] And although the findings of this practitioner do at first appear to be positive and worthy of attention, his conclusions are still tentative and will require more extensive follow-up studies involving a larger sampling of drug users.

Half-way Houses

Perhaps one of the best-known and most successful methods of treating drug abusers is the half-way house. The first half-way house was Synanon, founded in 1958 by Lewis Yablonsky. Although Synanon differs in some ways from other residential centers, such as Phoenix House or Topic House, many of its underlying principles and philosophical concepts are the same.

1. Ex-addicts are staff members.
2. Drug use of any sort is prohibited.
3. A person is admitted to the program only after having proved, through a series of stress/marathon sessions with other members of the community, that he or she is genuinely motivated to alter drug-taking behavior.
4. Once accepted into the community, the new member is expected to give the program his or her *total* attention.
5. After detoxification (without the aid of methadone) the new member is assigned to a work program—usually consisting of tasks of a menial nature.
6. Treatment consists primarily of group interaction and mutual reinforcement.
7. Increasing freedoms and privileges are contingent upon conformity.[5]

Essentially, the program involves four stages. The first stage is reached when the addict decides to join and comply with the rules of the community. If the addict can manage to abstain from using drugs and if he or she chooses to remain in the program, the addict is said to have entered the second stage. This stage is characterized by an extended period of self-reflection and self-evaluation, usually lasting from three to six months. During this period, the addict may experience severe depression, and is frequently overwhelmed by the horrors and waste wrought by the personal tragedy of his or her addiction. Naturally, the support of the community becomes vital at this time. The next stage occurs approximately one year after the addict has entered the community; to successfully complete this stage, the individual must make an even greater commitment to self understanding. The final phase comes six months to one year thereafter, and is marked by an emotional stabilization and a significant attainment (internalization) of behavioral controls.[6]

The major differences between Synanon and other residential therapeutic community centers revolve around the use of professionals and the period of treatment. Synanon, for example, has traditionally refrained from using professionals, whereas other centers employ professionals either as therapists or as advisors (usually members of the board of directors). Synanon also attempts to have its residents remain within the community for an indefinite period of time, encouraging them either to work or live in a Synanon-related facility. Other programs, in contrast, specify a certain time period during which the addict must undergo treatment.

Despite their respective differences, all the half-way houses have been subjected to a number of criticisms. Many contend that the treatment period is too long and that the staff involved is too extensive to effectively accommodate large numbers of addicts. Moreover, many question the long-term success of these programs. In the case of Synanon, for example, evaluation of the program has not always been entirely accurate. Investigators have noted that a major problem with the positive outcome rates (that is, the number of addicts who did not return to drugs after leaving the program) is that they fail to take into account the large number of addicts dropped or lost from the program during the early stages of treatment.

Civil Commitment

Another major approach to treating drug addicts, which is currently being used in both New York and California, is the civil commitment approach. Although this approach employs a number of therapeutic techniques, including both individual and group counseling, it is unique because of the manner in which addicts are recruited into the program. In this approach, an addict who has been arrested

> can choose to stand trial or enter a rehabilitation program lasting about three years. If the addict does not choose to enter the program and is found guilty while standing trial, the authorities in California and New York will probably send him to the rehabilitation-oriented program despite his original objection.[7]

An addict who is admitted to one of these programs is first detoxified, if necessary, and then sent to a rehabilitation center (sometimes this facility is a sort of modified prison); later, the addict is released to a half-way house, or is placed in a supervised aftercare program. Although in theory this approach is fairly comprehensive, some researchers question the whole concept of civil commitment.[8] If it could be shown to be effective as a means of "curing" heroin or cocaine addicts, it might not be an issue, but because it has not yet been proven successful, its value is being seriously questioned. Furthermore, many view civil commitment—which may not help the addict at all—as nothing more than a ruse in which the courts attempt to remove addicts from society under the guise of offering them treatment.

Methadone Maintenance

Methadone maintenance was especially welcomed as an approach to treating addicts since psychotherapy and punishment by incarceration seemed to have little impact.[9] This factor, coupled with the belief that addiction could ostensibly be treated as a medical problem, led to the establishment of several methadone maintenance programs in the hope that they might succeed where other approaches had not. Through the use of methadone, an antinarcotic agent capable of blocking the euphoric effects of heroin for long periods of time, they felt that the addict might be given a chance to completely conquer addiction and to eventually become reintegrated into society.

Inpatient and Outpatient Treatment

The original methadone maintenance program was established by Drs. V. P. Dole and M. E. Nyswander in New York City.[10] This program required that the addict be hospitalized for a period of six weeks. During this drug-free period, the patient received methadone on a regular basis, and was given psychological support as well as encouragement to explore educational and vocational opportunities through discussions with counselors.

Shortly after the establishment of this program, which was considered to be successful, a number of outpatient programs were initiated so that the methadone maintenance concept could be expanded to include more addicts. Some of these outpatient programs experimented with allowing patients to control their own methadone dosage. These techniques were referred to as "knowledge of dosage" and "methadone self-prescription."[11] Addicts participating in these experiments were either allowed to know the dosage of methadone they were on, or were given limited power to reduce or increase their own dosage. Surprisingly, most of the addicts participating in the experiments tended to *lower* their dosage. This trend seemed to indicate that the addict might be able to assume responsibility for self-administration of methadone. As Stern, Edwards, and Lerro report,

> since the methadone-on-demand technique seemed to avoid pathological confrontations by placing the major onus of treatment on the addict himself, and since this inclusion of the addict in the treatment planning has the effect of appealing to his maturity rather than to the regressive and childish aspects of his personality, we believe there is reasonable justification for this approach to detoxification.[12]

Another aspect of methadone maintenance outpatient programs is that many of them have sought to further ensure the rehabilitation of the addict by offering a number of other services in addition to the methadone treatment. These services include individual and group therapy, crisis intervention, family therapy, medical care, legal services, vocational guidance, and occupational placement.

The addition of these services came about in an attempt to capitalize on the use of methadone and, perhaps more important, to help minimize some of the problems that often accompany the use of a narcotic antagonist. As Ramer and his associates note, "receiving methadone brings about major disruptions in the (the addict's) life, and these disruptions require swift, supportive, and wise treatment."[13]

Pros and Cons of Maintenance

Despite its considerable success, methadone use has long been the target of strong negative criticism. On the positive side, a number of studies have reported that not only can methadone help addicts lead productive lives, but that it also has an indirect impact on the crime rate.[14] This is not surprising because once an addict is completely rehabilitated, he or she no longer needs to commit crimes to obtain money to support the drug habit.

On the other hand, the fact that methadone is itself an addicting drug, which produces withdrawal symptoms upon its discontinuation, leads many critics to speculate about the validity of its use. Among the most frequently heard arguments are the following:

1. Methadone maintenance is not a cure, but merely a process in which one addicting drug is used to replace another.
2. Methadone seals the fate of the individual who is only experimenting with heroin by literally forcing the person into addiction.
3. Methadone has no impact on the antisocial traits exhibited by some addicts and can (and often does) end up being illegally diverted onto the street.
4. Methadone overdose is possibly even more difficult to treat than heroin overdose, and may in some cases lead to death.
5. Methadone maintenance programs largely ignore the underlying causes of drug abuse, and tend to be concerned only with eliminating the symptoms.

Finding a New Solution

All of the approaches to treating alcoholics and drug addicts described in this chapter have been shown to have definite limitations. Of course, when one examines the criteria used to evaluate their effectiveness, or considers the prohibitive costs involved in conducting these various programs, it becomes easy to understand why so few of them have been successful.

Another possible explanation for the ineffectiveness of these approaches is that most of them are founded on philosophies that are either oversimplistic or that fail to take into account all the factors that contribute to drug abuse. Many of them are simply outmoded. A good example of such a philosophy is reflected in the following comment by Dr. G. E. Vaillant, in which he states that addicts should be encouraged in their efforts to find "the best possible dependency object, to sustain employment via external support, and to discover a more mature way to deal with his instinctual needs than solitary gratification."[15]

Clearly, a job and a growth experience are simply not enough. If they were, then those programs that provide occupational preparation and professional counseling would have a high rate of success. Even methadone maintenance programs, which, despite their shortcomings, have perhaps the highest success rates, still do not know how or where to direct addicts once they have overcome their dependence on heroin.

Thus the major problem in finding an effective means of treating alcoholics and drug addicts seems to lie in the fact that simply not enough is known about the underlying causes of serious drug abuse. In addition, what *is* known about drug abuse has yet to be integrated in such a way that research can be directed toward finding the important answers and ideas that are so desperately needed. The fact is that current efforts to treat drug addicts are, for the most part, without any sound, comprehensive theory to guide them. And this problem is only intensified by the fact that society is in a constant state of change. In light of what we now know, it would be unrealistic to expect significant results from present-day treatment programs. However, if we are to eventually be able to combat the ever-growing problem of drug abuse, we must continue to search for new and better solutions.

Notes

1. A. Lazerson, ed., *Psychology Today: An Introduction* (Del Mar, Calif.: CRM Books, 1972, pp. 676–677.
2. C. J. Rowe, *An Outline of Psychiatry* (Dubuque, Iowa: Brown, 1975), p. 158.
3. R. J. Wicks, *Correctional Psychology* (San Francisco: Canfield Press, 1974), p. 17.
4. T. E. Bratter, ''Group Therapy of Affluent, Alienated, Adolescent Drug Abusers: A Reality Therapy and Confrontation Approach,'' *Psychotherapy: Theory, Research and Practice* 9 (1972): pp. 308–313.
5. M. S. Cherkas, ''Synanon Foundation—A Radical Approach to the Problem of Addiction,'' *American Journal of Psychiatry* 121 (1965): pp. 1065–1068.
6. E. L. Markoff, ''Synanon in Drug Addiction,'' in J. H. Masserman, ed., *Handbook of Psychiatric Therapies* (New York: Science House, 1966), pp. 297–308.
7. R. J. Wicks, *Applied Psychology for Law Enforcement and Correction Officers* (New York: McGraw-Hill, 1974), p. 105.
8. J. C. Kramer, K. A. Bass, J. E. Berecocken, ''Civil Commitment for Addicts: The California Program,'' *American Journal of Psychiatry* 125 (1968): pp. 816–824.
9. V. P. Dole, M. E. Nyswander, and M. J. Kreek, ''Narcotic Blockade,'' *Archives of Internal Medicine* 118 (1966): pp. 304–309.
10. V. P. Dole and M. E. Nyswander, ''A Medical Treatment for Diacetylmorphine (Heroin) Addiction,'' *Journal of the American Medical Association* 193 (1965): pp. 646–650.
11. P. F. Renault, ''Methadone Maintenance: The Effects of Knowledge of Dosage,'' *International Journal of the Addictions* 8 (1973): pp. 41–48; H. V. Angle, S. Parwatiker, ''Methadone Self-prescription by Heroin Addicts in an Inpatient Detoxification Program,'' *Psychological Record* 23 (1973): pp. 203–214.
12. R. Stern, N. B. Edwards, and F. A. Lerro, ''Methadone on Demand as a Heroin Detoxification Procedure,'' *International Journal of Addictions* 9 (1974): p. 876.

13. B. S. Ramer, M. O. Zaslove, and J. Langan, "Is Methadone Enough? The Usage of Ancillary Treatment During Methadone Maintenance," *American Journal of Correction* 127 (1971): p. 1043.
14. R. T. Dale and F. R. Dale, "The Use of Methadone in a Representative Group of Heroin Addicts," *International Journal of the Addictions* 8 (1973): pp. 293–308; J. H. Jaffe, M. S. Zaks, and E. N. Washington, "Experience with the Use of Methadone in a Multi-modality Program for the Treatment of Narcotics Users," *International Journal of the Addictions* 4 (1969): pp. 481–490.
15. G. E. Vaillant, "A Twelve-year Follow-up of New York Narcotic Addicts: Some Characteristics and Determinants of Abstinence," *American Journal of Psychiatry* 123 (1966): p. 583.

Selected Bibliography

Accerri, F., and Blum, M. "Methadone Maintenance Bibliography." *Journal of Drug Issues* 4 (1974): 181–194.

Baganz, P., and Jarvis, J. "Work and Study Release in the Rehabilitation of the Narcotic Addict." *Rehabilitation Literature* 32 (1971): 354–359.

Baldridge, P.; McCormack, M.; Thompson, L.; Zanow, A.; and Primm, B. J. "Providing Incentives to Successful Methadone Patients—Experimental Program." *New York State Journal of Medicine* 74 (1974): 111–114.

Berecochea, J. E., and Sing, G. E., Jr. "The Effectiveness of a Halfway House for Civilly Committed Narcotics Addicts." *International Journal of the Addictions* 7 (1972): 123–132.

Berger, M. "Methadone Maintenance Programs." *Postgraduate Medicine* 54 (1973): 165–166.

Blanchy, P. H. "Recent Developments in the Therapy of Addictions." *Current Psychiatric Therapies* 12 (1972): 98–103.

Blane, H. T. *The Personality of the Alcoholic*. New York: Harper & Row, 1968.

Blum, E. M., and Blum, R. H. *Alcoholism*. San Francisco: Jossey-Bass, 1967.

Cahalan, D. *Problem Drinker*. San Francisco: Jossey-Bass, 1970.

Canada, A. T., Jr. "Methadone Treatment of Heroin Addicts." *Journal of the American Medical Association* 219 (1972): 910–911.

Carroll, C. *Alcohol Use, Nonuse, and Abuse*. Dubuque, Iowa: Brown, 1970.

Conrad, H. T. "Newer Treatment Approaches for Drug Addiction." *Medical Arts and Sciences* 25 (1971): 15–32.

Doctor, R. M., and Sieveking, N. A. "A Comparison of Attitudes Among Heroin Addicts, Policemen, Marijuana Users, and Nondrug Users About the Drug Addict." *International Journal of the Addictions* 8 (1973): 691–699.

Dole, V. P. "Detoxification of Sick Addicts in Prison." *Journal of the American Medical Association* 220 (1972): 366–369.

Freedman, D. X., and Senay, E. C. "Methadone Treatment of Heroin Addiction." *Annual Review of Medicine* 24 (1973): 153–164.

Glaser, F. B. "Gaudenzia, Incorporated: Historical and Theoretical Background of a Self-help Addiction Treatment Program." *International Journal of the Addictions* 6 (1971): 615–616.

James, I. P. "The Compulsory Treatment of Narcotic Addicts." *British Journal of Addiction* 67 (1972): 123.

Joseph, B. S. "Management of the Addict." *New England Journal of Medicine* 285 (1971): 971.

Joseph, B. S. "Lessons on Heroin Abuse from Treating Users in Vietnam." *Hospital and Community Psychiatry* 25 (1974): 742–744.

Karkus, H. D. "Methadone vs. Psychotherapy in the Treatment of Heroin Addiction." *International Journal of the Addictions* 8 (1973): 427–434.

Kissin, B., and Sang, E. "Treatment of Heroin Addiction, Multi-modality Approach." *New York State Journal of Medicine* 73 (1973): 1059–1065.

Lewis, E., Jr. "A Heroin Maintenance Program in the United States." *Journal of the American Medical Association* 223 (1973): 539–546.

National Institute of Mental Health. *Alcohol and Alcoholism.* Chevy Chase, Md.: NIMH, 1969.

Newcombe, J. "Treatment of Drug and Alcohol Dependence." *Lancet* 1 (1973): 491–493.

O'Brien, J. S.; Raynes, A. E.; and Patch, V. D. "Treatment of Heroin Addiction with Aversion Therapy, Relaxation Training and Systematic Desensitization." *Behaviour Research and Therapy* 10 (1972): 77–80.

Oppenheim, G. B.; Wright, J. E.; Buchanan, J.; and Biggs, L. "Outpatient Treatment of Narcotic Addiction—Who Benefits?" *British Journal of Addiction* 68 (1973): 37–44.

Perkins, M. E., and Wolkstein, E. "Methadone Maintenance: A Future for the Addict." *Journal of Rehabilitation* 39 (1973): 34–36.

Phillipson, R. "Drug Abuse Treatment." *Journal of School Health* 42 (1972): 625–628.

Pillard, R. C. "Shall We Allow Heroin Maintenance?" *New England Journal of Medicine* 288 (1973): 682–683.

Platt, J. J., and Labate, C. *Heroin Addiction: Theory, Research, and Treatment.* New York: Wiley-Interscience, 1976.

Popham, R. E., ed. *Alcohol and Alcoholism.* Toronto: The Addiction Research Foundation (University of Toronto Press), 1970.

President's Commission on Law Enforcement and Administration of Justice. *Task Force Report: Drunkenness.* Washington D.C.: U.S. Government Printing Office, 1967.

Raynes, A. E., and Patch, V. D. "An Improved Detoxification Technique for Heroin Addicts." *Archives of General Psychiatry* 29 (1973): 417–419.

Reeder, C. W.; Kunce, J. T.; Niewoehner, G. J.; and Inskeep, R. B. "Vocational Rehabilitation of the Hardcore Addict." *Rehabilitation Literature* 34 (1973): 11–14.

Renner, J. A., and Rubin, M. L. "Engaging Heroin Addicts in Treatment." *American Journal of Psychiatry* 130 (1973): 976–980.

Schut, J.; Wohlmuth, T. W.; and File, B. A. "Low-Dosage Methadone Maintenance: A Re-examination." *International Journal of Clinical Pharmacology* 7 (1973): 48–53.

Schut, J.; Wohlmuth, T.; and File, K. "High-dose Methadone Maintenance: An Evaluation." *British Journal of Addiction* 68 (1973): 145–150.

Seixas, R. C., and Eggleston, S. *The Person with Alcoholism*. New York: New York Academy of Sciences, 1974.

Smithers Foundation, Inc. *Understanding Alcoholism*. New York: Smithers, 1968.

U.S. Department of Health, Education, and Welfare. *First Special Report to the U.S. Congress on Alcohol and Health*. Washington, D.C.: Department of Health, Education, and Welfare, 1971.

Chapter 9

Enforcement and Prevention

Today, the area of drug abuse that commands the greatest amount of attention from legislators and criminal justice agencies is narcotics abuse. In recent years, the use of dangerous narcotics (once confined largely to urban ghetto areas) has become visible in all levels of society, making it one of the most serious issues confronting modern-day law enforcement agencies. Thus, this chapter will be primarily concerned with legislation and preventive measures geared toward the control of narcotics, although peripheral attention will also be given to some of the other major drugs of abuse.

Legal Measures Taken to Control Narcotics Abuse

Generally speaking, the war against narcotics abuse has been waged on three levels: international, federal, and state. The first major antinarcotics laws were enacted at the international and federal levels; these in turn set the stage for (as well as parallel) the overall development of the state laws.

International Narcotics Control: A Brief History

To gain an understanding of the impact of and progress made in antinarcotics laws, one should first know something about international efforts to enact narcotics control legislation. In the past, attempts to limit the distribution and use of narcotics have produced explosive results. Two wars between China and Great Britain, triggered to some extent by arguments over China's opium trade, bear this out. Indeed, international attempts at controlling narcotics traffic have been largely ineffectual because of a number of factors, including national self-interest and a general sense of apathy. This trend becomes apparent when one examines the outcome of several of the major historical meetings conducted on the international level to discuss the opium problem.*

---

*For a complete examination of the development of international antinarcotics policies and legislation, see J. J. Platt and C. Labate's *Heroin Addiction: Theory, Research, and Treatment* (New York, Wiley-Interscience, 1976).

Shanghai Conference—1909 The Shanghai meeting was important in that it represented the first formal international conference convened to discuss the opium problem. The United States hoped to gain commitments from foreign nations to limit opium growing and opiate exportation through enactment of stringent laws. The outcome of the conference, however, was disappointing. The general apathy as well as the lack of power invested in the representatives present at the meeting prevented the enactment of internationally sanctioned laws that would control narcotics traffic. The general consensus of the conference, however, did support the position that unbridled production and distribution of morphine and its derivatives should be curbed. And this recommendation in turn spurred the United States to take action in the form of legislation, and set the stage for subsequent informal international meetings, including a second international conference (Hague Conferences: 1912–1913), which resulted in the issuance of a statement recommending a number of steps aimed at narcotics control.

First Geneva Conference—1924 The United States hoped to secure the enactment of uniform international legislation that would succeed in curbing opium traffic and heroin production. By the end of the first Geneva conference, however, no decision to control morphine, cocaine, or heroin production had been reached; the lack of agreement resulted in a subsequent conference in Geneva, which also proved to be largely unproductive.

Conference on Limitation of Manufacture of Narcotic Drugs—1931 The outcome of the important 1931 meeting was the development of an elaborate system to regulate international narcotic production and manufacture. However, heroin production was still permitted rather than totally prohibited, as several of the delegates had proposed. The long-term effects of these impressive efforts to suppress illegal narcotics traffic are questionable.

Following the above conferences there were a number of other official gatherings which lead to major decisions pertaining to drug trafficking. Among the most successful of these conferences were:

1. San Francisco Conference of the United Nations—1945
2. Paris Protocol—1948
3. Opium Limitations Protocol—1953
4. Single Convention on Narcotic Drugs (United Nations)—1961

The measures enacted by these conventions and conferences failed to result in the appreciable curtailment of narcotics traffic and manufacturing that their proponents had hoped for. As a result, the United States proposed in 1972 that the Single Convention on Narcotic Drugs be amended so that an investigation of a nation's narcotics production might be undertaken should any question arise concerning the validity of its reports to the United Nations. Also, the United States suggested that action be taken against a nation involved in unreported, unauthorized narcotics activities which were previously discovered, and not rectified after the fact.

These recommendations by the United States seem to be an exercise in hopeful naiveté; nations will probably not allow a U.N. committee to audit their narcotic production until they are ready and willing to take all measures to curb their production, at which time an audit would become unnecessary.

Whether steps to completely curb narcotic production can be expected by every nation is questionable. At least, one can safely say that until all countries reach a point where they are encountering a drug problem themselves, they won't be willing to launch an all-out war on narcotics manufacturing and trafficking. Until that time, the United States can only do what is diplomatically possible to encourage other countries to at least attend to the problem in some meaningful way in their respective lands, and to act simultaneously to enforce its own federal laws, so that a model is set up for other nations to follow when they choose to do so.

Federal Legislation

Just prior to the first international conference on the opium problem held in Shanghai in 1909, the United States formulated a series of federal laws designed to curb indiscriminate narcotics use. These laws—and the ones that followed shortly thereafter—were prompted by a number of factors:

1. The desire to demonstrate to the world that it had exemplary drug laws.
2. The conviction that, as an international trend setter in the area of narcotics regulation, it could logically offer assistance to China which was having an opium problem; the United States wanted to establish better relations with China for economic and political reasons.
3. The belief that international restriction in the manufacture and exportation of opiates was needed if the nation's narcotic problem was to be dealt with effectively.
4. The absence of any established federal restrictions on the importation of crude opium was a current issue that had to be dealt with.
5. The existence of a flourishing drug industry that was involved in the sale of patent medicines having an unknown opiate content and an unpublished list of ingredients.
6. The fear that minority groups might revolt while under the influence of an addicting narcotic.
7. A means to allow druggist and physician groups the opportunity to gain power and recognition through involvement in drafting regulations that would explicitly permit them to maintain control of drug dispensing and implicitly establish them as the professional caretakers of legal drug use.

Between 1903, when the American Pharmaceutical Association's ad hoc Committee on the Acquirement of the Drug Habit was convened, and the time when the Treatment Act of 1972 was enacted, a number of efforts were made to curb drug abuse in the form of recommendations, laws, and rulings. (See Table 9.1.)

Defining the Issues If anything, the legal provisions of these acts, and the recommendations that resulted from professional meetings on the problem of drug abuse, demonstrated that there was a great deal of confusion surrounding the subject. Accordingly, there were many unanswered questions which elicited many varied tentative answers in the form of ever-changing laws and viewpoints. Do narcotics have medicinal value or should they be banned? Is drug addiction a disease and a medical problem, or is it a symptom of criminality? Should an addict be punished or treated? Which is the most important area of focus, enforcement or rehabilitation? If the addict is to be treated, how should this be accomplished and by whom? Could a physician treat an addict on an outpatient basis? If so, should the physician be able to prescribe maintenance doses or progressively smaller doses? On the other hand, if addiction cannot be effectively treated, should there not be a series of severe mandatory penalties to deal with addicts and those involved in the manufacture or transportation of narcotics?

Breakthrough Legislation Many of the difficulties involved in answering these questions, and in turn in providing appropriate federal legislation, are still being debated. However, one of the most recent major drug acts does appear to demonstrate a clearer understanding of at least some of the dimensions of the current drug problem. The Comprehensive Drug Abuse Prevention and Control Act of 1970 (Public Law 91–513) contains provisions stating that penalties for drug offenses must be determined on the basis of such factors as the type of drug, whether it was a first offense, whether the person was a user or a seller, and whether the person convicted was a minor or had sold to a minor. The significance of this act is that it represented a basic recognition of the obvious difference between a person convicted of continued heroin use and someone found guilty on a first offense for marijuana possession.

TABLE 9.1 PERTINENT PROVISIONS OF KEY ACTS AND COMMITTEE RECOMMENDATIONS ON DRUG CONTROL: 1903–1970

1. American Pharmaceutical Association ad hoc Committee on the Acquirement of the Drug Habit (1903)
   The committee recommended:
   1. Severe penalties for illegal drug sale.
   2. Strong state enforcement of laws.
   3. Eliminate *all* opium importation.
   4. Unrefillable heroin prescriptions be issued only by a physician.
2. Pure Food and Drug Act (1906)
   There was one noteworthy provision in this act:
   1. Patent medicines traded in interstate commerce must provide labeling of any narcotic content.

3. Harrison Act (1914)
   This act had several significant provisions:
   1. Records have to be kept of drugs received by addicts from registered physicians.
   2. Revenue stamps required on packages containing more than the permitted amount of opiates and records of transactions involving retail sales of them; severe penalties for violation of these provisions.
   3. Registration with Internal Revenue Collector of agents involved in opiate manufacture, sale, or transportation.
4. Webb et al. v. United States (1919)
   Supreme Court Ruling: Outlawed addiction maintenance.
   Behram v. United States (1922)
   Supreme Court Ruling: Outlawed *any* prescription of narcotics for addicts.
5. Narcotic Drug Import and Export Act (1922)
   By this act, severe penalties (fine of not more than $5,000 and ten years in prison) were instituted for a narcotics conviction.
6. Linder v. United States 268 U.S. 5 (1925)
   Supreme Court Ruling: Physician could prescribe narcotics in moderate dosage to relieve withdrawal symptoms.
7. Uniform Narcotic Act (1932)
   This act was designed to coordinate federal and local record keeping of drug transactions.
8. Narcotics Drug Control Act (1956)
   This act imposed severe penalties for drug-related offenses.

Offense	Penalty
Possession, 1st	2 to 10 years
Possession, 2nd	5 to 10 years (mandatory sentence)*
Selling, 1st	5 to 10 years (mandatory sentence)*
Possession, 3rd	10 to 40 years (mandatory sentence)
Selling, 2nd	10 to 40 years (mandatory sentence) or possibly death sentence if seller is over the age of 18 and if the sale is to a minor.

9. American Medical Association and American Bar Association Joint Committee on Narcotic Drugs (1958)
   The Committee recommended experimental outpatient treatment for addicts; less provision for severe penalties.
10. Robinson v. United States 370 U.S. 660 (1962)
    Supreme Court Ruling: Addiction should not be punished by imprisonment, except in those cases where civil commitment for treatment is refused.
11. Comprehensive Drug Abuse Prevention and Control Act (1970)
    1. Superseded all other federal narcotic laws.
    2. Bureau of Narcotics and Dangerous Drugs (BNDD) was given enforcement powers over drugs controlled by the act.
    3. Penalties based on drug classification, whether it is a first or subsequent offense, and type of involvement (that is, possession, sale, manufacture).
    4. Severe penalties for anyone convicted of sale of narcotics to a minor.
    5. Leniency for first offender.

*Mitigating circumstances cannot be taken into account by the court.

Title II of this act was called Control and Enforcement. It is also known as the Controlled Substance Act (CSA). The CSA contains the control mechanisms by which the federal agencies responsible for drug enforcement of the act determine the effects of controlling a substance covered by it. (See Table 9.2.)

The Drug Enforcement Agency (DEA) and the Food and Drug Administration (FDA) share responsibility for enforcement of the CSA. They are both concerned with the CSA's control over production, sale, and procurement of the substances controlled under the act.

Through systematic registration of persons authorized to possess substances under the CSA (that is, manufacturers, wholesalers, importers, researchers, physicians, hospitals, and pharmacies), dealers in controlled substances are able to determine whether a customer can legitimately receive them simply by checking with the DEA, which maintains a list of all authorized buyers. If this verification process is not followed and/or inadequate steps are taken by the dealer to prevent release of controlled substances into unauthorized hands, loss of one's registration can result and permission to be a legitimate drug dealer can be revoked.

Unauthorized sale or distribution of controlled substances is also discouraged by the requirement in the CSA for maintenance of a thorough record-keeping system covering the possession and transfer of controlled substances. (There are exceptions for medical doctors and persons involved in research.) This record keeping becomes especially important in the case of those substances listed in Schedules I and II because of a government-determined quota (established by DEA and FDA) which limits the production of substances falling into these categories to the approximate amount of legal drug usage estimated for them.

In addition to procedures related to registration, record keeping, and quotas, there are six other types of control mechanisms affecting substances listed in the CSA. The control devices involve restrictions on distribution and dispensing, export and import limitations, provisions for drug storage, reports of transactions, and criminal penalties for illicit trafficking.

In regard to distribution, a dealer must receive a DEA-issued order form from a customer before transferring Schedule I and II drugs to the customer. Although no order form is needed for Schedule III, IV, and V drugs, distribution is restricted in these cases by holding the dealer responsible for verifying customer registration numbers against the files at the DEA before releasing any controlled substance to them.

Dispensing controlled substances again depends upon the schedule to which it applies.

Schedule I: These drugs can be distributed by an established number of manufacturers only to authorized researchers who will be administering the substances directly to their subjects.

Schedule II: These drugs are supplied only upon presentation of a written, non-refillable prescription that is signed by a physician.

Schedules III and IV: These drugs are supplied upon presentation of a written prescription or made up in response to a doctor's call, with limited refill provisions, which can be further limited by the physician.

Schedule V: These drugs are distributed to persons aged 18 and over, who have sufficient identification. A log is maintained by pharmacists of the names of persons to whom they supply over-the-counter drugs in this category.

The import and export restrictions of substances under the CSA vary primarily in the following way: The DEA must approve any international transfer of Schedule I and II drugs and be given prior notice as to the import and export of Schedule III, IV, and V substances.

Security for storage of substances controlled under the CSA differs as one might expect. Schedule I and II drugs require high security (that is, a 24-hour alarm system and a specially constructed vault) whereas security for substances listed in the other schedules is much less stringent. Retail suppliers of controlled substances are not subject to the same security requirements as manufacturers, importers, and wholesalers; to require small dealers to provide similar security would be impractical.

The last two control mechanisms involve the established systems in which drug transfers are to be reported to DEA, and the criminal penalties for illegal trafficking. (See Table 9.2.) One of the most significant aspects of the CSA is that it contains a provision that clearly distinguishes between drug abuse and drug sale. Drug abuse is indicated when the person convicted clearly needs treatment; drug sale applies to large-scale sellers who need to be incarcerated and put out of circulation. In this sense, the CSA is particularly advanced over many of the acts that preceded it—which is saying a lot, considering the long history of acts that have been passed at the federal level over the years.

State-level Legislation

While the list of federal antinarcotic laws enacted since 1906 reflects a long-standing concern on the part of Congress and the executive branch of the government with the nation's drug problems, state legislative actions represent at least an equal commitment to and concern with drug abuse in the United States. The state of California enacted the first anti-opium statute as early as 1872. And, in fact, some of the states had already passed drug acts by the time of the initial passage and enactment of a federal drug-control bill.

Understandably, drug-control statutes have varied—often markedly—from one state to another. And it was not until 1970 that the Uniform Controlled Substance Act was adopted with the goal of bringing state laws in line with federal drug legislation. Attesting to the importance of the need for a coordinated legislative approach to the drug problem is the fact that many states have already passed this act with only minor revisions.

TABLE 9.2 COMPARISON OF THE SCHEDULES OF THE CONTROLLED SUBSTANCES ACT (CSA) IN TERMS OF CONTROLS IMPOSED

SCHEDULE*	TYPES OF SUBSTANCES COVERED (PARTIAL LIST)	RECORD KEEPING	MARKETING QUOTAS	DISTRIBUTION RESTRICTIONS
I	Heroin, LSD, mescaline, psilocybin-psilocyn, MDA, marijuana, hashish, hashish oil	Records must be kept separate from all other records of the handler (for easy audit)	Yes	DEA order form required prior to transaction
II	Opium, morphine, meperidine, methadone, methaqualone, cocaine, phenmetrazine, methyl phenidate			
III	Glutethimide, some amphetamines, narcotics, stimulants, and depressants, DCP	Records need not be separated but must be kept in a readily retrievable form	No, but some drugs limited by Schedule II Quotas	DEA registration number required
IV	Chloral hydrate, meprobamate, some stimulants, and depressants			
V	Over-the-counter drugs containing codeine and certain narcotics			

*Registration is required with DEA for handlers of substances in all schedules.

<table>
<tr><th></th><th>DISPENSING LIMITATIONS</th><th>IMPORT/ EXPORT</th><th>SECURITY REQUIRED</th><th>MANUFACTURER/ SUPPLIER RE-PORTS TO DEA</th><th>CRIMINAL PEN-ALTIES FOR TRAFFICKING (FIRST OFFENSE)</th></tr>
<tr><td>I</td><td>For research only</td><td>Permit re-quired from DEA</td><td rowspan="2">High secur-ity (i.e., spe-cial vault, 24-hour alarm)</td><td rowspan="2">Yes</td><td rowspan="2">Narcotic: 15 years/$25,000
Nonnarcotic: 5 years/$15,000</td></tr>
<tr><td>II</td><td>Written, signed, unrefillable pre-scription required</td><td></td></tr>
<tr><td>III</td><td>Written or phoned-in pre-scription refillable up to 5 times in 6 months if so authorized by physician</td><td rowspan="2">Permit re-quired from DEA for nar-cotics; prior notice to DEA of planned transporta-tion involv-ing nonnar-cotics</td><td rowspan="2">Special security (i.e., surveil-lance)</td><td>Yes, for narcotics</td><td>5 years/$15,000</td></tr>
<tr><td>IV</td><td></td><td>No</td><td>3 years/$10,000</td></tr>
<tr><td>V</td><td>I.D. required—cannot be a minor</td><td>Permit re-quired for import of narcotic prepara-tions; prior notice re-quired for export of narcotics and import/ export of nonnar-cotics</td><td></td><td>Yes, for manufac-turers of narcotic preparations</td><td>1 year/$5,000</td></tr>
</table>

SOURCE: Drug Enforcement Administration: *Fact Sheets* Washington, D.C.: U.S. Government Printing Office, 1973).

Another trend that is almost uniform in nature is the move away from classifying marijuana users and first offenders as continual drug abusers. Less severe penalties for marijuana use and dismissal of charges made against a first offender if the offender fulfills a long-term probationary period without incident are becoming the accepted procedure in most states.

However, despite the general move toward adoption of the Uniform Controlled Substances Act and less severe penalties for certain types of drug users in special circumstances, there are states which still mete out harsh penalties.

If statutes and their enforcement are to be effective, the states whose laws are in sharp contrast to the Uniform Controlled Substance Act will eventually have to alter them. For when they do so, cooperation between federal, state, and local agencies involved in law enforcement will be made easier. This is especially important since each level of government must be involved in narcotics enforcement if illegal drug trafficking is to be controlled. To expect optimum results while there are still marked differences between state and federal laws, which in turn imply different enforcement procedures, is not only unrealistic but also practically impossible.

Today, persons in both the private and government sectors of society are deeply concerned with the enforcement issues surrounding the use of dangerous drugs. Community interest and action are widespread and diversified. Medical, mental health, and legal professionals as well as clergy, educators, parents, students, and concerned citizens are joining law enforcement professionals in the search for a practical and effective solution to the growing drug problem.

Private Narcotic Enforcement Agencies

Within the private sector numerous organizations have sponsored research projects aimed at obtaining information on drug abuse. And as one might expect, nongovernmental criminal justice associations have been particularly active in this area. Written material, meetings, consultant services, and other types of assistance related to narcotic and drug abuse are currently available from such organizations as the International Association of Police Chiefs, the National Council on Crime and Delinquency, and the National Sheriffs' Association. One private organization that is particularly devoted to providing information on drug abuse to criminal justice officers is the International Narcotic Enforcement Officers' Association.

International Narcotic Enforcement Officers' Association*

Law enforcement officers and professionals in related fields are expected to have a knowledge of the various drugs of abuse, the laws concerning them, and

*International Narcotic Enforcement Officers' Association, 178 Washington Avenue, Albany, New York 12210

modern techniques of drug investigation. Unless they have this knowledge, their work in the area of narcotic education and enforcement will be seriously hampered.

Given this urgent need for information pertaining to drug abuse, it became clear that what was needed was a private organization whose primary concern would be narcotic enforcement, an organization that could provide opportunities for an ongoing exchange of views on issues related to the narcotics problem. This need was realized by many law enforcement officers and narcotic agents as early as the late 1950s, at which time the drug problem was fast becoming a major health and crime issue. By 1960, the stage was set for the formation of a new organization. All that was needed was the right person to head a broad-based group. This person turned out to be Dr. John J. Bellizzi, the man who was finally responsible for forming the International Narcotic Enforcement Officers' Association (I.N.E.O.A.).

Dr. Bellizzi, who has had professional experience in narcotic enforcement work and who has a broad educational background in law, chemistry, and pharmacology, is not only a highly respected lecturer on drug abuse but has also served as a consultant to the Commission of Narcotic Addiction in New York City and the White House Conference on Narcotics and Dangerous Drugs.

The I.N.E.O.A. has come a long way since 1960 when Dr. Bellizzi first assembled twenty-five representatives from various enforcement agencies at a meeting held in Albany, New York. Today the association includes narcotic enforcement officers from all levels of government and many medical, research, pharmacological, university, and drug industry personnel. It has representatives from every state in the United States, from every province of Canada, from every country in South America, and from over fifty other nations throughout the world. Through its annual conferences, it has brought together legislative, administrative, medical, psychological, and law enforcement professionals, educators, and personnel from the pharmaceutical industry to share their views on the problems of narcotics abuse.

The International Narcotic Enforcement Officers' Association is a testimony to the interest of private citizens in curbing the use of dangerous drugs. Efforts such as these are particularly important in that they parallel and reinforce government work in this vital area.

Public Narcotic Enforcement Agencies

Combating drug abuse is a complex task involving input from municipal, county, state, and federal enforcement agencies. Local and state efforts vary so widely from region to region and from department to department that it would be almost impossible to make any general comments on the nature of their work or the extent of their effectiveness. However, one point can be made with some degree of certainty. When agencies begin to cooperate with one another and pool their efforts, they almost invariably become more effective. But once they allow themselves to become more concerned with who will receive credit for a given arrest than with the overall objectives of the cooperative effort, they will become considerably less effective. The fine work of the metropolitan enforcement groups (MEGS) bears this out.

An appreciation of the value of cooperation and unification of efforts can be seen on the federal level as well. Indeed, it was precisely this recognition of the need for coordination that gave rise to the creation of the Drug Enforcement Administration and the Special Action Office for Drug Abuse Prevention.

Drug Enforcement Administration (DEA)*

Within the past decade, the United States has experienced a national health crisis that has touched upon every stratum of American society. This crisis is drug abuse. To combat this overwhelming problem, the federal government mobilized an all-out effort, with the Drug Enforcement Administration (DEA) at its vanguard. The primary objective of this new agency is to halt illicit trafficking in narcotics and dangerous drugs. The Drug Enforcement Administration was created on July 1, 1973, by congressional approval of a presidential reorganization plan.

Prior to the establishment of the DEA, governmental efforts to combat the abuse of narcotics and dangerous drugs had been divided among several different federal agencies, each pursuing its own independent course of action.

To provide leadership for a concentrated, worldwide attack on narcotics trafficking and drug abuse, the presidential reorganization plan specified that the Bureau of Narcotics and Dangerous Drugs, the Office for Drug Abuse Law Enforcement, the Office of National Narcotics Intelligence, the drug investigative and intelligence units of the Bureau of Customs, and the drug enforcement sections of the Office of Science and Technology should all work together under the auspices of the DEA.

Enforcement In the enforcement of drug laws, the major emphasis is placed on the source and distribution of illicit drugs rather than on the arrest of drug abusers. The DEA is thus primarily concerned with arresting the flow of drugs at their original foreign sources, disrupting illicit domestic commerce at the highest levels of organization, and assisting state and local police in preventing illegal drugs from reaching the community.

To accomplish these goals, the DEA is responsible for the development of an overall federal drug strategy through workable programs, planning, evaluation, and intelligence. The DEA is also charged with full investigation and preparation for prosecution of suspected violators of federal drug laws, and conducts relations with law enforcement officials of foreign governments under the policy guidance of the Cabinet Committee on International Narcotics Control.

*Source for this section: Drug Enforcement Administration: *Fact Sheets* (U.S. Government Printing Office, Washington, D.C., 1973), pp. 3–5.

To perform its mission the DEA has stationed highly trained agents in major cities throughout the United States as well as in forty-five offices in thirty-one countries throughout the world. The objectives of DEA agents are to reach the highest possible source of supply and to seize illicit drugs before they reach the abuser. To achieve this goal, they combine advanced enforcement techniques with the use of modern technology and equipment.

The Drug Enforcement Administration is also responsible for the regulation of the legal manufacture of drugs and other controlled substances under the Controlled Substances Act of 1970. Under this act the DEA is required to establish import, export, and manufacturing quotas for the various controlled drugs. Physicians, pharmacists, and other persons who handle, dispense, or prescribe controlled drugs are subject to periodic inspections by DEA representatives. These controls ensure an adequate supply of legal drugs for medicine and research and at the same time prevent the possibility that these drugs might be diverted into illegal traffic.

Intelligence An efficient intelligence operation is vital to the success of any law enforcement agency. The DEA has its own Office of Intelligence, which is staffed by experienced criminal investigators and intelligence analysts. Every DEA Regional Office in the United States and in foreign countries has its own Regional Intelligence Unit. All information concerning individuals or organizations involved in trafficking in narcotics and dangerous drugs is furnished to the Office of Intelligence, where it is compiled, analyzed, and disseminated in the form of a finished intelligence product.

This information provides personnel in the Office of Enforcement with important intelligence data that will enable them to attack the drug traffic at its most vulnerable source. It also provides the administrator and other government agencies with strategic intelligence information influencing policy decisions, deployment of resources, and overall strategy. Intelligence on shifts in the drug traffic, the types of drugs being abused, and the effectiveness of foreign and domestic programs are all part of this intelligence process. Another important facet of the DEA intelligence program is that it promotes an ongoing exchange of information between federal, state, local, and foreign law enforcement agencies.

Training The National Training Institute of the DEA offers intensive training programs in narcotics and dangerous drugs for law enforcement officers from agencies throughout the United States and the world. Ten-week sessions are conducted in which police officers receive training that is similar to that which DEA special agents receive. In addition to intensive practical instruction in drug-law enforcement techniques, they are introduced to management concepts that will enable them to develop and lead drug investigative units. Specialized two-week schools offer eighty hours of instruction to state, county, and city officers in the basic techniques of narcotics and dangerous drugs investigation. These schools are held at the DEA's National Training Institute in Washington and at field locations throughout the country.

The DEA has recently intensified its efforts in the area of international training. The National Training Institute now conducts intensive practical-training programs in foreign countries. These programs are designed to satisfy the needs of the recipient nation as well as to assist the Administration in its international enforcement mission. Ranging in length from two weeks to one month, these programs are conducted in the native language of the participant and are heavily reinforced with practical exercises that utilize the most sophisticated enforcement techniques and equipment available. The DEA also conducts practical training programs in several languages for selected police officials of foreign nations. These schools offer extensive instruction in drug-law enforcement techniques and intelligence gathering, and train participants to effectively lead the efforts of cooperating nations in the international drug interdiction effort. Qualified English-speaking officers can also participate in ten-week police training schools. Special seminars and briefings are conducted for forensic chemists, other federal agencies, civic groups, foreign dignitaries, and other visitors to the United States.

Scientific Research In an attempt to accumulate up-to-date information pertaining to the drugs under its jurisdiction, the DEA encourages controlled scientific research in the area of drug abuse. The Administration's research is confined to gathering information that will assist law enforcement agencies in their efforts to combat the drug abuse problem. It encompasses the clinical, social, psychological, and biological aspects of drug abuse. As part of its scientific staff, the DEA employs physicians, pharmacologists, chemists, statisticians, pharmacists, and professional educators.

Another function of the DEA is performed by its Science Services Division, which is responsible for administering the six regional laboratories and the Special Testing and Research Laboratory that are part of the DEA laboratory system. Regional laboratories are operated in New York, Washington, D.C., Miami, Chicago, Dallas, and San Francisco. The Special Testing and Research Laboratory is located in McLean, Virginia.

Virtually all controlled substances cases require physical evidence for their successful prosecution. It is the primary function of these laboratories to provide definitive identification of such substances, and to provide expert testimony in court. Much of this evidence can also be of value to law enforcement agencies who are attempting to establish drug-traffic patterns. These laboratories also provide in-depth analyses of evidence, and have facilities for fingerprint processing, photographic processing, and photographic printing and development.

Prevention Programs Drug abuse prevention is another responsibility that belongs to the Drug Enforcement Administration. As part of its program to make citizens aware of the hazards of narcotics and dangerous drugs, the agency provides factual information in the form of literature, speakers, films, and displays to a variety of organizations. The DEA also works closely with educators, local, state, and national government agencies, law enforcement officials, and organizations in planning and conducting abuse prevention programs. Efforts are made to conduct these activities at the regional level whenever possible.

Law Enforcement Assistance Cooperation between all levels of enforcement agencies has been a key factor in the planned attack on narcotics trafficking. DEA agents actively assist state and local police through task forces and metropolitan enforcement groups (MEGS). These task forces concentrate their enforcement efforts on organizations or individuals engaged in drug trafficking within specific regions. To a large extent, they rely upon the cooperation of local police departments in the areas of planning, intelligence, and enforcement.

Special Action Office for Drug Abuse Prevention*

The federal government first recognized the existence of a drug problem in this country over sixty years ago. Early government response, embodied in the Harrison Narcotic Act of 1914, was directed almost exclusively at controlling the supply of dangerous drugs. The Harrison Act established federal control over the supply, distribution, and use of narcotic drugs in the United States, imposing strong legal penalties for illicit possession or sale of narcotics. But almost no attention was given to the treatment and rehabilitation of drug users until the early 1930s, when the U.S. Public Health Service hospitals at Lexington, Kentucky, and Fort Worth, Texas, were established to treat drug addicts. By the mid-fifties many locally supported treatment programs had been established across the country.

The high rate of relapse by addicts after treatment indicated that a better understanding of the problems of rehabilitation, new methods of treatment, and far greater attention to prevention and education were needed. Throughout the 1960s, the federal government sponsored a number of research and experimental programs in the area of drug abuse. In 1967, the Office of Economic Opportunity initiated community-based programs for treatment and rehabilitation of addicts in poverty areas of the country's major cities.

By the end of 1968, a number of federal agencies were engaged in drug-abuse prevention activities, and more were entering the field. Some were concerned mainly with treatment and rehabilitation, others with research and education. Some agencies carried out programs themselves, and many gave financial support to projects operated by universities or private groups. It became

*Source for this section: Drug Enforcement Administration: *Fact Sheets* (U.S. Government Printing Office, Washington, D.C., 1973), pp. 63–66.

increasingly clear that until efforts could be coordinated at the federal level, it would be difficult to bring coherence to the growing number of programs operating under federal support.

Accordingly, in the late fall of 1970, then-President Richard Nixon created a White House task force of experts and consultants from outside the government to make recommendations on how the federal government might best utilize its resources to cope with the many problems of drug abuse. Acting on the recommendations of this task force, the president undertook to develop a single coordinating agency at the highest federal level. The Special Action Office for Drug Abuse Prevention was created as a result of this effort.

Dr. Jerome H. Jaffe, Chairman of the White House Task Force, was asked by President Nixon to become Director of the Special Action Office in the summer of 1971. He was replaced by Dr. Robert DuPont in June, 1973.

The Special Action Office for Drug Abuse Prevention was established by President Nixon under an executive order on June 17, 1971. The Special Action Office was created by the Drug Abuse Office and Treatment Act of 1972, which had the unanimous approval of Congress. The act was signed by the president on March 21, 1972.

The basic objectives of the Special Action Office were (1) to take immediate steps toward reducing drug abuse in the United States; and (2) to develop a comprehensive, long-term federal strategy to combat drug abuse. The president and Congress directed the Special Action Office to exercise broad authority to accomplish these vital tasks, but it was not authorized to fund or operate ongoing programs, although it could develop promising new concepts and approaches to problems of drug abuse. The director reported directly to the president.

The Special Action Office was in charge of all federal programs or activities relating to drug abuse education, training, treatment, rehabilitation, and research. Currently, there are nineteen federal departments and agencies engaged in the non-law enforcement aspects of drug abuse prevention. Seven are concerned with treatment, nine with rehabilitation, four with training, nine with education, four with evaluation, and seven with research. A major task of the Special Action Office was to coordinate the efforts of these various agencies, evaluate their performance in programs related to drug abuse, and work with them to improve services.

The long-term assignment of the Special Action Office was to analyze the nature, extent, and trends of drug abuse in the United States and to examine various approaches to solving the drug abuse problem in order to develop effective action programs. Most important, the Special Action Office set goals, established priorities, and specified how federal resources of funds, programs, services, and facilities could be used to combat drug abuse in the United States.

Priorities for the Special Office There are two major groups that are currently receiving urgent attention—heroin addicts who commit a significant portion of all urban crime, and the growing number of young drug abusers. Priorities for the work of the Special Action Office emphasized new initiatives in the field of drug abuse prevention and treatment.

Under the act which created the Special Action Office, the director had the following responsibilities:

1. To provide overall planning and policy, and to establish objectives and priorities for all federal drug-abuse prevention programs.
2. To review the regulations, guidelines, requirements, criteria, and procedures of operating agencies to assure compatibility with national drug-abuse prevention strategy.
3. To examine and evaluate federal legislation, budgets, and programs, and to recommend needed changes in organization, management, and personnel.
4. To develop and demonstrate more effective drug-abuse prevention programs.
5. To encourage and promote expanded research programs and clinical research facilities.
6. To coordinate federal programs with the drug-abuse prevention activities of state and local governments and public and private agencies and individuals, and to provide technical and professional assistance.
7. To foster drug-abuse prevention, treatment, and rehabilitation programs and services in state and local governments and in private industry.
8. To submit an annual report to the president on the activities of the Special Action Office.

The final responsibility of the Special Action Office was to make preparations for its own orderly phase-out by June 30, 1975, which was accomplished.

Progress Initiated under the Special Office Significant progress was being made toward dealing with drug abuse problems. Increased federal funds and new techniques to secure them have been approved to fight drug abuse. Since 1969, federal support has increased fourfold for research, sixfold for treatment and rehabilitation, and thirtyfold for education and training.

Treatment and rehabilitation continues as the first priority. Between June 30, 1971, and June 30, 1972, the number of federally funded treatment programs in operation increased from 135 to more than 320. Nearly 90 began operation in the last three months of fiscal year 1972. In terms of patients in treatment this meant an increase from 16,000 in June, 1971, to more than 51,000 on August 30, 1972, more than triple the original number. Expansion of treatment has resulted from close coordination between SAO and other agencies. It also reflects the development of more efficient start-up procedures by SAO. Fee-for-service contracts, keyed to cost and quality standards and targeted on geographical areas of greatest need, have been a major innovation.

The Special Action Office scrutinized the budgets and evaluated the policies of all civilian federal agencies engaged in drug abuse prevention, with the exception of those offices dealing with law enforcement. It worked with each agency to establish specific goals and to shape the budgets needed to achieve them. A system to monitor and evaluate these efforts was organized.

New programs were developed to reduce abuse among GIs in Vietnam, and at other bases overseas and at home. Military police has shifted to treat drug abuse as a medical problem rather than as a strictly disciplinary problem. A massive screening program has been set up to detect drug abusers, who are then provided treatment and rehabilitation services.

The Special Action Office helped conduct a nationwide review of all the methadone maintenance programs in the United States, and the status of the drug has been changed from a research tool to that of a recognized form of medical treatment administered under strict government controls. Increasing numbers of addicts are voluntarily seeking this treatment, and programs are being expanded to accommodate them.

With the help of the National Bureau of Standards, the Special Action Office developed a technique to prevent methadone from being diverted to illicit channels and to protect the anonymity of those under treatment. To reduce the possibility of diversion, a longer-lasting methadone is under development.

The Special Action Office expanded the education and training of those who are dealing with the nation's drug abuse problems, including teachers, medical personnel, and laymen. The National Drug Abuse Training Center established in Washington, D.C., trains people in the latest techniques of drug abuse prevention. Other federally supported centers train persons to teach new skills to others in their communities. Through the U.S. Office of Education, all fifty states are helped to strengthen their own drug abuse prevention efforts.

Through new grant programs operated by the National Institute of Mental Health, the Special Action Office assisted medical schools to expand their course work in drug abuse problems. Physicians and other medical professionals are being trained in the latest techniques for drug abuse diagnosis and treatment.

New technical assistance in combating drug abuse is being offered to the states. The Special Action Office assembled teams of professionals to help communities with special drug abuse problems and to set up demonstration programs. The National Clearinghouse for Drug Abuse Information is being expanded to offer the latest information in the drug abuse field to professionals and others. On request, the clearinghouse furnishes information on medical and educational techniques and offers suggestions on how to establish local drug abuse programs.

A master reporting system to collect data on all kinds of drug abuse is being organized. New programs have been started to gather information on the amount and patterns of drug abuse and to note shifts in trends of usage.

Because nearly half of all street crimes committed in the United States are thought to be drug-related, the Special Action Office developed a new concept in which arrested drug abusers were offered a number of treatment alternatives.

They were offered methadone maintenance and other forms of treatment to break the drug addiction-street crime cycle. In cooperation with the Law Enforcement Assistance Administration, the concept is being implemented in a number of metropolitan areas.

Research has been stepped up in a variety of drug abuse areas. New and more effective narcotics antagonists are being tested; simpler ways of screening for drug abuse are under development; studies are under way to determine the implications of long-term use of marijuana. Morphine and heroin are being restudied for possible physical dangers that may not have been recognized. New studies are being conducted to find out what motivates people to voluntarily give up drugs, and on educational techniques to prevent them from starting at all.

Looking Ahead Along with its mandate from the president and from Congress to control today's drug abuse epidemic "in the shortest possible time," the Special Action Office was also instructed to plan for the future. In this task, it provided the staff for the Strategy Council, established along with the Special Action Office under the 1972 Drug Abuse Office and Treatment Act.

The council is a permanent group made up of heads of the key federal agencies responsible for drug abuse programs. It aided the Special Action Office in the development of long-range federal policy on drug abuse and was responsible for continuing that policy after the phase-out of the office.

The council ties together the health and medical aspects of drug abuse programs with the law enforcement efforts to eliminate illicit drug supply and traffic. It operates on the principle that law enforcement must be coupled with a rational public health effort to prevent drug abuse and to detect, treat, and reclaim the drug abuser.

With the help of the Special Action Office, the council encouraged all Americans to join in the fight against drug abuse, not only doctors, scientists, nurses, and teachers, but parents, students, businessmen, and citizens from all walks of life. It asks all parts of the community—churches, schools, civic groups, and businesses—to mobilize their resources for effective action.

Selected Bibliography

Anonymous. "History of Heroin." *Bulletin on Narcotics* 5 (1953): 3–16.

Ball, J. C., and Chambers, C. D., eds. *The Epidemiology of Opiate Addiction in the United States*. Springfield, Ill.: Thomas, 1970.

Levine, H. R. *Legal Dimensions of Drug Abuse in the United States*. Springfield, Ill.: Thomas, 1974.

McNamara, J. D. "The History of United States Anti-opium Policy." *Federal Probation* 37 (1973): 15–21.

Musto, D. F. *The American Disease: Origins of Narcotic Control*. New Haven: Yale University Press, 1973.

Platt, J. J., and Labate, C. *Heroin Addiction: Theory, Research and Treatment*. New York: Wiley-Interscience, 1976.

Simmons, L. R. S., and Gold, M. B. ''The Myth of International Control: American Foreign Policy and the Heroin Traffic.'' *International Journal of the Addictions* 8 (1973): 779–800.

Strategy Council on Drug Abuse. *Federal Strategy for Drug Abuse and Drug Traffic Prevention*. Washington, D.C.: U.S. Government Printing Office, 1973.

Tennyson, A. L. ''History and Mechanism of International and National Control of Drugs of Addiction.'' *American Journal of Medicine* 14 (1953): 578–585.

Chapter 10

Criminal Investigation and Drug Abuse

A number of comprehensive works on criminal investigation and interrogation interviewing have already been published. It is beyond the scope or intent of this chapter to examine these topics as thoroughly as some of the books that are listed in the bibliography. However, there are a number of specific investigative problems related to crimes involving drug abuse that do merit mention here.

Drug Abuse in the Community

Usually, investigators assigned to drug abuse cases are already quite familiar with general investigation techniques. Even so, many of them still admit to having special difficulties in using investigative techniques in cases involving illegal drug sale, use, and transportation. It is therefore not surprising that in addition to a thorough knowledge of investigative techniques, drugs, and drug laws affecting investigations and case build-up, narcotics agents and detectives must also be resourceful and persistent if they are to be successful.

Ideally, drug abuse investigators must be able to function in unusual and demanding circumstances. As investigators or as undercover agents, they have to be able to:

1. Effectively develop and employ sources of information such as informants.
2. Imaginatively conduct a surveillance in difficult situations.
3. Carefully plan and execute raids and individual arrests.
4. Methodically search persons and property for drugs and related equipment.
5. Efficiently collect and preserve evidence.

Accordingly, drug-abuse investigative work needs to be carried out by persons who are efficient, personally and professionally motivated, and, if possible, able to easily fit into the "current drug scene." Fitting into the "current drug scene" means speaking, acting, and playing an inconspicuous role in the area of the operation when the circumstances require.

Sources of Information

Information in an investigation of drug abuse can be gathered from various sources. The most frequently used are informants and community sources such as businesses and government agencies.

Informants The use of informants is essential in investigating drug abuse cases. Although *total* reliance on intelligence information received from informants should be avoided, developing and employing sources of information is an important aspect of the drug investigation work of the narcotics agent and the detective.

To help remove the stigma that has been attached to the employment of informants in the past, some federal agencies are teaching their trainees to classify informants as "sources of information." They feel that informant use should be seen in the same positive light that other information sources are because of the overall value of this technique. In contrast to the disdain that once surrounded the use of a "squealer," "rat," or "informer," modern criminal justice agencies are teaching investigators how to cultivate these valuable and important sources of information.

Many agencies hold periodic conferences at which officers can present profiles of new informants in order that other agents, who might have dealt with similar types of individuals in the past, can offer advice. At these conferences, protection of the identity of the informant is also discussed—it is important that the informant's cover not be compromised or his or her safety jeopardized; the fact that the topic of informant safety is discussed at all is reflective of the new attitude toward the positive use of informants.

Informants can provide a number of services to undercover agents. These include the following:

1. Getting information on drug caches, names of dealers, and areas of operation.
2. Introducing the officer to street sellers and on rare occasions to upper-echelon dealers.
3. Giving the agent "street acceptance" by being seen together.
4. Gathering information that can be recorded and used in future investigations.
5. Helping the agent to determine the size and configuration of the area's major drug operations.

Sources of information may agree to assist agents for any number of reasons, but primarily they do so for money, revenge, or clemency. Addicts and former addicts are often willing to provide information in return for cash payment. They may not divulge their own source of narcotics or provide an introduction or lead to a major dealer, but they can help the agent gain acceptance into a portion of the drug scene.

Revenge against a competitor—usually another small-time drug seller—or a dealer who has cheated them is another motive leading addicts to supply information. A third frequent reason for complicity with the law is a desire for clemency after being arrested on a drug or robbery charge.

This cooperation, however, is limited in scope. Officers who fail to realize this may put too much trust in their informants. This misplaced confidence in the informant can result in a double cross, injury to an officer, theft of drug "buy money," or even possible loss of an agent's life.

Extreme caution should be exercised in the use of informants. Accordingly, agents need to recognize the practicality of setting up a number of guidelines for themselves in the use of informants to prevent unnecessary problems.

1. Continually evaluate the reliability of informants' reports; don't accept information on face value as being valid. (Consider the reason why they are providing the information, as well as the source and details of the material being presented.)
2. Be careful not to promise a payment that can't be made.
3. Use informants only when necessary.
4. Limit the amount of information they are provided to only what they need to know to carry out their instructions.
5. Provide detailed instructions, and have informants repeat them to demonstrate their complete understanding of the operation and the limits of their involvement in it. (Informers should not be instructed to commit a crime or act in a supervisory role or coordinate any part of the operation.)
6. When informants report in, question them methodically and in detail to make certain that they haven't left anything out.

If sensible guidelines such as these are followed, informants as sources of information can be most valuable. The undercover agent can gain a good deal of information on drug-trafficking operations and be introduced into the drug scene.

Other Sources Although informants are extremely valuable in investigating the use, sale, or transportation of drugs, narcotics officers need to realize that there are other valuable sources of information as well. Business people from the community, police records, public agencies and records, and private corporations (for example, the telephone company) can supply a good deal of information to drug agents. (Check the bibliography at the end of this chapter for books on investigative techniques.)

In surveying the information gleaned from other noncriminal sources of information (whether unsolicited from a person or a written report), investigators sometimes fail to be critical enough in their evaluation of such information. What they tend to forget is that even the most well-meaning person may be biased in some way. Therefore, even the comments received from noncriminal sources must be carefully interpreted by the investigator. Drug use is an emotional issue today; people have strong feelings about drug abuse in general, and users and sellers in particular. Therefore, when evaluating and utilizing their comments, the agent must continually try to separate what informants know from what they believe or feel to be correct.

In essence, the thumb rule in employing *any* source of information is: Use informants, but use them with caution.

Surveillance

Surveillance is another difficult but necessary function that drug abuse investigators must perform. Without proper surveillance, potentially valuable information can easily be lost. By observing the actions of an alleged dealer or by following the actions of an undercover agent who is due to make a big buy, corroborating evidence of a crime can frequently be obtained and, in some circumstances, potential harm to an agent whose cover has been compromised can be averted.

Surveillance may also result in attaining information which can: (1) aid in uncovering the working patterns of a drug operation; (2) establish a basis for a search warrant request; and (3) generally provide further leads that may culminate in a raid on a building where drug supply, manufacturing, or use is taking place.

Physical surveillance of a suspect is especially difficult in drug cases. Being familiar with the geographical area as well as the physical appearance of the suspect is helpful. Use of many agents (in vehicles and on the street), electronic devices, and neighborhood informants can make the job easier. But the experienced street agent provides a better method because he or she can blend into the neighborhood and move about naturally. The agent's maneuverability is often the crux of the operation. If the agent can observe a series of transactions between a dealer and an undercover agent or other buyers, information can be gathered for current prosecution and also for securing a future case.

Planning an Arrest/Raid

Prior to a raid or a street arrest or taking a major drug distributor into custody, considerable planning must take place. (Even when a law enforcement operation is quickly mounted to deal with an immediate situation, unless time is allotted for coordination, the overall effectiveness of the raid may be greatly diminished.) As a result, the chief investigator should know the answer to a number of questions before giving permission to agents to conduct a raid or drug arrest.

1. Do the agents have the proper arrest and search warrants?
2. Will enough officers be available?
3. Do agents know the roles they are supposed to play during and subsequent to the raid?

4. Is everyone familiar with the physical layout of the area and with the resistance expected?
5. Does the case in question warrant a raid at this particular time? (In other words, is there sufficient reason to believe that the operation will net as many of the parties involved in the drug ring as possible? Based on current knowledge of the extent of the involvement of the suspects to be arrested, it must be determined that a raid at this time will not preclude the arrest of a more important figure.)
6. Are the officers who are not involved in the post-raid search aware of their functions? (See below.)

Once the raid has taken place and the suspects have been advised of their rights and taken into custody, a number of steps need to be taken by those officers not involved in the actual search of the premises. The suspects need to be carefully searched, needle marks (if present) photographed, and various medical tests conducted (urine, blood, and so forth) to determine whether narcotics have recently been used. Investigators remaining at the crime scene have the responsibility of conducting a more extensive search.

Conducting the Search

A methodical approach, persistence, and imagination are needed to conduct an effective search of persons, crime scenes, vehicles, and narcotic storage areas in drug abuse cases. In conducting these searches, officers are looking for drugs, related equipment for drug processing, and pertinent information which might further the investigation, such as records of sales, addresses of buyers, and lists of pickup and drop-off points.

There is no substitute for a knowledge of the physical appearance and types of packaging of the commonly abused drugs. In addition, it is advantageous for officers to be aware of the types of paraphernalia associated with the various drugs, and the materials employed in illegal drug processing.

Although only a partial list, the following items are examples of the types of materials an investigator might encounter and be expected to collect during a drug search:

Forms of Drugs

Gelatin capsules (heroin)
White powder (heroin/cocaine)
Leaf, usually having 5 to 7 serrated blades (cannabis)
Greenish-brown tobacco (marijuana)
Brown powder, usually in block form or wrapped in small packets (hashish)
Tablets, cubes, gum, foil packets, or vials (LSD)
Legally manufactured drugs in tablet, capsule, liquid, or suppository form (barbiturates, amphetamines)

Equipment Used in Drug Use, Manufacture, and Transportation

Bent seared teaspoon and/or cap
Tourniquet (large rubber band or elastic belt)
Eyedropper, syringe, cotton, glassine bags, paper, and needles (all used to prepare heroin or cocaine for injection)
Pipes—regular and water—are often used to smoke marijuana and may contain residue
Ash tray—may contain marijuana ashes
Laboratory equipment
Scales
Transportation devices (for example, hollow-walled luggage)

Because an investigator must be on the lookout for so many different objects and substances when searching persons and property in drug abuse cases, such searches are usually difficult and time-consuming. Knowing where to look does not make the job easier, but it does decrease the chances that an officer might overlook something important.

There are no shortcuts in searching persons and property; a good search must be methodical and complete. An officer doesn't find a packet of narcotics in a drain merely by accident—a good deal of hard work is involved. The investigator must know where and what to look for and be willing to take the time to do it. (See Tables 10.1, 10.2, and 10.3. When searching a suspect's premises the investigator must be methodical and imaginative, even more so than when conducting a search of a person or a vehicle. Accordingly, Table 10.3 contains suggestions and is not meant to be comprehensive.)

TABLE 10.1 AREAS OF DRUG CONCEALMENT TO BE CONSIDERED WHEN CONDUCTING A SEARCH OF A PERSON

Capsule hidden in hair	Socks
In or under wig	Shoes
Inside or taped behind ears	Cuffs
Nose	Ties
Under tongue	Handkerchief
Under false teeth	Underside of belt
Under loose filling in tooth	Belt buckle
Swallowed with string attached to tooth	Inside trousers
Glass eye	False buttons
Taped under breast	Wallet
Rectum	Tobacco pouch
Vagina	Inside paperback book
Between toes	Inside handbag (check contents as well as the lining of the handbag itself)
Taped to bottom of feet	Eyeglass case
Hat lining	Pens
Jacket lining/lapels	Inside sanitary napkins or tampons
Shirt pockets/lapels	Under bandaids
Collar stays	In any packages/umbrella being carried

TABLE 10.2 AREAS OF DRUG CONCEALMENT TO BE CONSIDERED WHEN CONDUCTING A SEARCH OF A VEHICLE

Taped under hood/truck	Glove compartment
In engine area (for example, air or oil filter)	In hollowed-out steering wheel
Behind headlights or taillights	Under horn
Hubcaps	In/under seats
License plate	Roof light
Bumpers	In detachable shift nob
Underside of car	Under pedals
Attached to gas cap	Under/in sun visors
Trunk bed/trunk contents	Cigarette lighter
Attached to inside of tires or inside spare tire	Speakers
Under rugs	In/behind radio/tape deck
Behind doors	In/under arm rests
Ashtrays	In loose contents of car (for example, packages, items in glove compartment)
	Behind dashboard
	Under window stripping

TABLE 10.3 AREAS OF DRUG CONCEALMENT TO BE CONSIDERED WHEN CONDUCTING A SEARCH OF ONE'S PREMISES

In/under furniture	Shutters and curtains
Rugs	Heating and air-conditioning units
Plumbing	Appliances
Wall and ceiling fixtures and moldings	Hanging outside the window, in the toilet bowl tank, and so forth
Telephones	In toys
Books	Inside/between magazines and newspapers
Decorations	Medicine cabinet and its contents
Foodstuffs	Cooking utensils
Hollowed-out wooden objects (for example, doors, bookcases)	Closets
Fishtanks	Clothes
Flower pots	Lamps
	Records and tapes

In conducting any type of property search investigators must have the tools and materials they need to get into, under, and around furniture, plumbing, appliances, flower boxes, and so forth. Such equipment might include:

Flashlights or droplights
Knife and scissors
Tweezers
Claw hammer, wrenches, and screwdrivers
Garden claw and small shovel
Measuring tape
Camera
Straightened wire hangers
Twine

Although these tools might make the search more efficient, they will not necessarily cut down on the amount of work involved; a properly conducted search in drug cases requires time and thoroughness if it is to be successful.

The Legal Search When officers conduct a search that turns out to be illegal, their efforts to develop a criminal case based on the evidence collected will be in vain. As a result, knowing what constitutes the requirements for a legal search is quite important. Generally speaking, a search is considered legal if it is conducted within the following guidelines:

1. Investigators obtain a legal search warrant.
2. The search is conducted within the reach of the suspect being arrested.
3. The search is conducted with the free, clear, and full consent of a suspect who is also fully aware of his or her constitutional rights.

There have been instances where officers have tried to get around these restrictions, but usually they resulted in the case being thrown out of court, or in the courts' becoming more critical of police searches.

There is simply no way to avoid the hard work involved in—as well as the legal limitations of—conducting a search. Once investigators realize this, a good deal of frustration over prosecution and court actions in pending drug cases can be avoided.

Physical Dangers There are always certain dangers involved in investigating a drug abuse case. An informer may "turn bad," a major dealer may become suspicious, or a street agent's cover may be compromised, resulting in the injury or death of the agent. An addict or seller may violently react and injure an investigator who is off guard during a raid.

In addition to dangers posed by persons involved in the abuse, sale, manufacture, or transportation of illegal drugs, considerable harm can also be done to investigators who inadvertently inhale chemicals or who improperly handle drug substances and paraphernalia during the course of a search. For example, contaminated needles can transmit infectious hepatitis if the agent's skin is broken by it in the process of picking it up. Some chemicals and drugs may produce an undesirable effect or cause damage to the body if inhaled or handled without gloves.

Consequently, care should always be taken when searching persons, vehicles, and property to avoid unnecessary harm. Such precautions should include the following:

1. Substances discovered should never be inhaled or handled without gloves, but should be sent to the laboratory for analysis.
2. All chemicals should be treated as though they were potentially combustible or caustic.
3. Ventilation of an area in which a laboratory is in operation should be effected immediately upon discovery until a member of a crime lab can be called in to shut off the equipment.

4. If a drug is accidentally handled or the investigator's skin is pricked with a needle, the skin should be washed thoroughly and medical attention obtained as soon as possible.

Collecting Evidence

To ensure that the evidence that is found is available for use in court, the investigators must carefully collect, mark, package, and systematically file receipts for the material that is uncovered in a search. More often than necessary, fingerprints on drug containers and the original state of the evidence found are lost due to improper handling or failure to maintain a complete system of receipts. To minimize the loss of material that may be used as evidence, a number of guidelines should be followed.

1. Original containers with suspected drug substances in them should be collected, recorded, marked, and placed in a secure envelope. This is done so that (a) none of their contents is lost; (b) they are retained in their original state; and (c) they can be identified by the person who found them.
2. Paraphernalia and residue (for example, in ashtrays) should be collected and secured in the manner described above.
3. Any drugs and packets found wrapped should be left intact and placed in a secure envelope or bag. (Aluminum foil is sometimes used as a wrap for LSD to protect it from exposure to light.)
4. Ashes and bags which may have contained drugs should also be collected and preserved in the manner noted for other types of evidence listed above.
5. Descriptive notes should be made on all evidence collected. They should only refer to the substances in terms of quantity, color, shape, size, and so on, since chemical analysis is needed to conclusively determine the nature of the substance.
6. Once narcotics are sealed, an identification tape should be attached to the envelope, which includes at least the officer's name, lab destination, case number or code name, and suspect's name.
7. A record of who has possession of confiscated drugs should be continually maintained. A receipt for the evidence should be signed by the person taking the drug to the lab, and a record of future changes in possession should be recorded until the material is entered as evidence in court.

Important and relevant evidence that is not properly collected, packaged, or receipted may prove to be useless to a prosecutor. This point needs to be continually made—especially to novice investigators—for material that has lost its evidentiary value through mishandling costs criminal justice personnel much unnecessarily wasted time and effort.

Use of Field-test Kits Once suspected drug substances are collected they are usually sent to a crime laboratory. Such laboratories have the facilities to reliably analyze the drugs and to provide complete identification of all substances.

In some instances time is a crucial factor in analyzing a substance for drug content. A central laboratory serving several counties may be overloaded with analysis requests. An undercover agent who has just made a "buy" or parents who are worried about their son's strange behavior may bring to the lab substances which they suspect to be narcotics. In these instances quick analysis is necessary to determine whether the substances are, in fact, drugs. If a local lab cannot provide immediate assistance, a field test is often performed.

Field tests of suspected drug substances are made with commercially produced kits. The number of different drugs that can be detected by these devices and the overall reliability of the tests varies greatly. Some of them, however, are capable of detecting the presence of heroin, cocaine, barbiturates, amphetamines, and marijuana in a substance.

After obtaining literature on field kits and reviewing their use by other criminal justice agencies, many law enforcement departments have instituted limited use of them. Although the kit may save time, the instances in which positive identification of a drug is missed—either through human error or inherent limitations in the kit in detecting certain kinds of drugs—make it advantageous to send unknown suspected drugs to a lab whenever possible. Therefore, field-test kits are recommended only for limited use.

Combating Drug Abuse in the Community

From the above discussion of utilizing sources of information, conducting a surveillance, executing a raid, searching for drugs, and properly collecting and field-testing drug substances, it should be evident that investigating drug abuse cases represents considerable work for the agents involved. Employing correct methodology, understanding and applying proven undercover techniques, and keeping abreast of new drug laws and related issues will help the investigator, but will not reduce the number of working hours he or she must devote to combating drug abuse. Drug abuse investigation in the street is one of the most demanding activities that can be undertaken by a criminal justice agent. The agent who accepts this fact before embarking on drug work will be well on the road to being an effective narcotics investigator.

Drug Abuse in Correctional Institutions

Drug abuse in the free community presents a mammoth investigation problem to criminal justice agents. Unfortunately, this problem doesn't end once the drug user is incarcerated, for illegal drug use in correctional institutions is also a problem today.

The actual size of the problem, however, is still undetermined. Some correction officials say the drug traffic is minimal or nonexistent in their institution or system. But a number of ex-offenders have privately claimed that it is easier to get drugs in jail than it is on the street. The truth probably lies somewhere in between. In the past, evidence has been uncovered indicating that certain jails and prison facilities do have a major drug traffic problem; inmates did have easy access to both soft and hard drugs. Furthermore, even though a particular correctional facility may not have a drug traffic problem at the present time, steps should be taken to prevent its developing one in the future.

Security officials in penal institutions usually have difficulties in controlling contraband. Since the introduction of drugs into the prison community is always a potential problem, officials must continually be on their guard. Correctional administrators need to keep informed and to be aware of such basic issues concerning drug control in the institutional setting as methods of entry, distribution and payment for drugs, investigation techniques and problems, and preventive measures.

Methods of Entry

Reducing the flow of contraband into correctional facilities is quite a challenging problem—especially in the case of drugs, which can be transported in any number of widely divergent forms and quantities. Drugs find their way into an institution in much the same manner that other types of contraband do. They can enter by mail or be brought in by visitors and employees.

Most institutions prohibit the receipt of packages by inmates unless they are items sent directly from the manufacturer or, if books or magazines, from the publisher. However, even with such precautions as these, drugs can still come through the mail in letters unless special care is taken to prevent such entry. A tab of LSD can easily be secured under a stamp or concealed in the cushion in a mechanical greeting card. Even the most stringent methods of mail control can't completely arrest the influx of drugs. Furthermore, if security measures become too strict, the exorbitant amount of time spent by correctional personnel to enforce them would reach a point of diminishing returns; such overbearing measures might also lead to a tense confrontation between prison officials and inmates, provoking an unnecessary riot.

Drugs are also often brought in by visitors, who then pass them on to the inmates. Searching the visitors is impractical, so a careful search of the inmates and their clothing should be made after each ''contact visit''—that is, one in which the visitor has physical access to the inmate.

The most frequently used method of drug entry into the institution is by means of employees. They have easy access not only to the interior area of the institution, but also to the inmate population. Therefore, distribution is quite easy for them.

Distribution and Payment

Once an employee brings drugs into the prison, they can be delivered to the intended individuals by direct distribution, by an inmate agent, or by leaving them at a prearranged drop point. Each method has its particular advantages. Direct distribution is the surest method, but it is also the one that involves the most risk. The dealer is sure that the right person is getting the drugs which have been brought in. Still, getting caught is highly possible since the user and the dealer are in direct contact at least once during the transaction.

Distribution to the inmate population by an agent is a very organized and usually safe method. However, giving power to an inmate agent can have special drawbacks. The agent may begin to pressure the dealer for a more profitable arrangement for himself after acting as the go-between several times. In addition, the agent may begin negotiating personally with the other inmates to obtain a greater profit for himself, causing possible discontent and ultimate exposure of the operation by a disgruntled user.

The safest method for the employee-drug dealer to use is to leave the drug consignment at a prearranged drop point. In this way a direct link to the drugs or the user is minimized for the dealer. Yet, the disadvantage is that the user can always claim that the drugs were taken by someone else before the pickup—which in some cases may actually be true.

Payment can take many forms and can be made inside or outside the institution. Inside the facility it can take the form of "contraband money" (actual cash which the inmate is not supposed to have while incarcerated), or possibly the promise of some service. The promise may be in the form of a pledge to do a job (robbery or assault, for example) upon release. It may also involve a promise not to reveal past criminal activities of the employee to superiors or to outside criminal justice authorities.

Payment on the outside can be of a similar nature. Moreover, sexual favors by an inmate's girlfriend or wife is one additional method of payment on the outside, which correctional investigators must be aware of.

Investigation

No matter what the method of payment or distribution, when drugs are used in a correctional setting, it will usually come to light eventually. In the case of employee-delivered drugs, the first hint of drug traffic is observed when rumors about illegal drug use begin to spread among inmates and employees. Such rumors may begin when an inmate receiving drugs starts to boast to others that he or she is able to get drugs and other prohibited material through "connections." Following these rumors, security and investigative follow-up procedures need to be stepped up in an effort to ascertain whether drugs are in fact being brought in by one or more of the employees.

Often, when there are continued rumors about inmate drug abuse, an inmate will approach the District Attorney or someone in the prosecuting branch of the criminal justice system. This inmate may approach the D.A. with the purpose of revenge (possibly he or she couldn't get drugs from the dealer), or to get special consideration for early release from jail in exchange for information or being involved in ''setting up'' the employee.

If the resulting investigation leads to the identity of the perpetrator, correctional officials frequently link up with outside law enforcement personnel to complete the operation. Working as a team, they may then take steps to put surveillance on the suspect in an effort to be in a position to observe the drug pickup and payment on the street, the employee bringing the drugs into the facility, and the distribution and payment inside the institution. With the aid of informants, chemically treated money, and numerous agents, the employee might be apprehended.

Problems in Investigation A number of things can go wrong in an investigation, however. In the above-outlined case of the employee who was under surveillance from the time of the drug buy to the point where the employee left the facility after being paid off with chemically treated money, any number of unforeseen events might have occurred:

1. The suspect may have spotted the surveillance soon after the buy and disposed of the drugs shortly thereafter.
2. A fellow employee may have tipped off the suspect, prompting the quick disposal of the drugs in one of several means.
3. The suspect may have sensed that the inmate betrayed him and aborted the sale at the last minute.

There are other problems that may arise during the course of the investigation as well. One of these involves the difficulties tied to the reluctance of many employees to report those they work with, even in instances in which they have reasonable proof of their implication in a drug-trafficking operation. This hesitation is especially evident when it comes to members of the uniformed force. Due to the comradeship in the ranks, informing on a fellow officer may be felt to be an act of disloyalty.

In such instances, the warden needs to remind the staff that an officer who deals in drugs endangers institutional security and places fellow officers in danger. Fights over the drugs brought in, unusual actions by inmates while under the influence of drugs, and the fact that the employee-dealer may be pushed into a position where he would have to bring in weapons to avoid being turned in by the inmate population all point to the need to report a dishonest employee. Furthermore, one of the roles of a criminal justice agency is to police itself. Unless this is done, its credibility will drop to the point where its effectiveness will be seriously questioned.

Another problem faced by correctional investigators is the safeguarding, handling, and marking of evidence by line personnel. In many systems, correction officers do not receive the same training in evidence preservation that police and peace officers on duty in the open community receive. Accordingly, material which might have qualified as evidence is ruled out as inadmissible because: (1) it wasn't marked and packaged in such a way that it could later be identified by the officer; or (2) it wasn't correctly receipted and stored, and an accurate record of the custodianship was not maintained.

To prevent this from occurring, a number of guidelines have been given to correction officers by their departments to help them know how to handle and preserve evidence. But many correctional systems still do not provide such guidelines or training in evidence preservation, resulting in an unnecessary loss of convictions in this area.

A number of guidelines should be followed when collecting and preserving evidence—including drug substances, preparation devices and other paraphernalia—found in a drug search.

1. Material found should be marked so that it can be identified later by the officer involved, packaged, and sealed.
2. Once packaged, an identification card should be attached to the package indicating the area in which it was found, the name of the officer who found it, and the person to whom it would be handed over; a record of the chain of possession should be created; and a receipt should be received by the officer from the person to whom the material is released (for example, the superior officer or lab technician).
3. When material is found in an institution, care must be taken to leave fingerprints intact by handling it as one would any potential evidence in a case; to photograph or sketch the area in which it was found (if a sketch is used, measurements should be taken); to list the names of any witness who may arrive on the scene at the same time; and to record a *description* of the item, without indicating any opinion on the item's nature (since this will be determined later by lab analysis).

Preventive Measures

In addition to continuing efforts to prevent the entry of drugs into the correction facility by monitoring the mails and searching inmates after contacts with visitors, there are a number of other steps which can be taken to prevent drug abuse resulting from the actions of a dishonest employee. One step is related to the proper orientation of civilian personnel; another action involves adhering to a departmental policy of dealing quickly and decisively with employees caught distributing drugs to inmates.

Civilian employees need to be apprised of the rationale behind existing security measures. A regular meeting should be held to discuss how inmates coerce employees to bring in seemingly harmless, but prohibited, items. By pointing out the harmful secondary value that a particular item has for an inmate, and by showing how the inmate can eventually press the civilian to bring in such things as drugs once he has him "hooked," employees can avoid becoming victims of circumstance. Preservice orientation and in-service classes on security for civilian employees are ideal times for this information to be disseminated.

Uniformed personnel also need to be continually reminded of the duty they have to "keep their own house clean." All rumors about an officer bringing in drugs need to be followed up. If the officer is innocent of illegal activity, then he or she should be cleared of suspicion by means of a thorough investigation. In those cases where evidence comes to light, officials must be motivated to pursue the investigation because they must realize that a dishonest officer puts fellow-officers in danger. An officer's disregard for the welfare of other officers should not be rewarded by their support of him. Potentially dishonest officers must be made to realize that once they begin to deal in drugs with the inmates, it will only be a matter of time until they get caught.

Drug control in a correctional institution is not an easy task. Established investigative procedures, an organized prevention program, and quick follow-up on initial signs of drug trafficking are sorely needed if the drug problem is to be controlled in the correctional setting.

Summary

Criminal investigation is a broad area in terms of both theory and practical application. The issues involved in conducting an investigation of a drug abuse case are as perplexing as they are unique.

In this chapter no attempt has been made to survey all aspects of criminal investigation; texts which do this are listed in the bibliography at the end of this chapter. What has been provided in this chapter is a brief coverage of those specific problems and techniques which an investigator might encounter in a drug case. Hopefully, this chapter has provided some indication of the intricacies and extensive work involved in investigating drug cases, and demonstrated how important it is for investigators to be properly trained, imaginative, motivated, and able to recognize the necessity of employing all the resources at their disposal.

Selected Bibliography

Aubry, A. S., Jr., and Caputo, R. R. *Criminal Interrogation.* Springfield, Ill.: Thomas, 1972.

Deinstein, W. *Techniques for the Crime Investigator,* 2nd ed. Springfield, Ill.: Thomas, 1974.

Fox, R. H., and Cunningham, C. L. *Crime Scene Search and Physical Evidence Handbook.* Washington, D.C.: U.S. Department of Justice, 1973.

Gerber, S. R., and Schroeder, O. Jr. *Criminal Investigation and Interrogation.* Cincinnati: Anderson, 1974.

Harney, M. L., and Cross, J. C. *The Narcotics Officer's Notebook.* Springfield, Ill.: Thomas, 1961.

Horgan J. J. *Criminal Investigation*. New York: McGraw-Hill, 1974.

Inbau, F. E., and Reid, J. E. *Criminal Interrogation and Confessions*. Baltimore: Williams & Silkins, 1967.

Levine, S. M. *Narcotics and Drug Abuse*. Cincinnati: Anderson, 1973.

O'Hara, C. E. *Fundamentals of Criminal Investigation*. Springfield, Ill.: Thomas, 1970.

Wicks, R. J. *Applied Psychology for Law Enforcement and Correction Officers*. New York: McGraw-Hill, 1974.

Wicks, R. J., and Josephs, E. H., Jr. *Techniques in Interviewing for Law Enforcement and Correction Personnel*. Springfield, Ill.: Thomas, 1972.

Appendix

Glossary of Technical Terms*

ADDICTION. In 1957, the World Health Organization (WHO) defined drug addiction as a state of periodic or chronic intoxication produced by the repeated consumption of a drug. Its characteristics include: (1) an overpowering desire or need (compulsion) to continue taking the drug and to obtain it by any means; (2) a tendency to increase the dose; (3) a psychic (psychological) and generally a physical dependence on the effects of the drug; (4) an effect detrimental to the individual and to society. (Compare with "drug dependence" and "habituation.")

ANALGESIC. Pain killer.

CENTRAL NERVOUS SYSTEM. The brain and spinal cord.

CONVULSIONS. An involuntary and violent irregular series of contractions of the muscles.

DELIRIUM. A condition characterized by mental excitement, confusion, disordered speech, and, often, hallucinations.

DEPRESSANT. Any of several drugs which sedate by acting on the central nervous system. Medical uses include the treatment of anxiety, tension, and high blood pressure.

DRUG DEPENDENCE. As described in 1963 by WHO, drug dependence is "a state arising from repeated administration of a drug on a periodic or continuous basis." Its characteristics will vary with the agent involved. This is made clear by designating the particular type of drug dependence in each specific case—for example, drug dependence of the morphine type, of the cocaine type, of the cannabis type, of the barbiturate type, etc. (Compare with "addiction" and "habituation.")

HABITUATION. As defined in 1957 by WHO, drug habituation is a condition, resulting from repeated consumption of a drug, which includes these

*From J. B. Williams, *Narcotics and Drug Dependence* (Beverly Hills, Calif.: Glencoe Press, 1974). Used with permission.

characteristics: (1) a desire (but not a compulsion) to continue taking the drug for the sense of improved well-being that it engenders; (2) little or no tendency to increase the dose; (3) some degree of psychic dependence on the effect of the drug, but absence of physical dependence and, hence, no abstinence syndrome; (4) a detrimental effect, if any, primarily on the individual. (Compare with "addiction" and "drug dependence.")

HALLUCINOGEN. Any of several drugs, popularly called psychedelics, which produce sensations such as distortions of time, space, sound, color, and other bizarre effects. While they are pharmacologically non-narcotic, some of these drugs (e.g., marihuana) are regulated under Federal Narcotic laws.

HYPNOTIC. An agent that induces sleep.

NARCOTIC. This term has two definitions. Medically defined, a narcotic is any drug that produces sleep or stupor and also relieves pain. Legally defined, the term means any drug regulated under the Harrison Act and other Federal narcotic laws. Some of these regulated drugs are pharmacologically non-narcotic (e.g., cocaine).

PHYSICAL DEPENDENCE. Physiological adaption of the body to the presence of a drug. In effect, the body develops a continuing need for the drug. Once such dependence has been established, the body reacts with predictable symptoms if the drug is abruptly withdrawn. The nature and severity of withdrawal symptoms depend on the drug being used and the daily dosage level attained.

POTENTIATION. Potentiation occurs when the combined action of two or more drugs is greater than the sum of the effects of each drug taken alone. Potentiation can be very useful in certain medical procedures. For example, physicians can induce and maintain a specific degree of anesthesia with a small amount of the primary anesthetic agent by using another drug to potentiate the primary anesthetic agent. Potentiation may also be dangerous. For example, barbiturates and many tranquilizers potentiate the depressant effects of alcohol.

PSYCHOLOGICAL DEPENDENCE. An attachment to drug use which arises from a drug's ability to satisfy some emotional or personality need of an individual. This attachment does not require a physical dependence, although physical dependence may seem to reinforce psychological dependence. An individual may also be psychologically dependent on substances other than drugs.

PSYCHOSIS. A major mental disorder; a serious mental derangement. "Psychosis" replaces the old term "insanity."

SEDATIVE. An agent which quiets or calms activity.

SIDE EFFECTS. A given drug may have many actions on the body. Usually one or two of the more prominent actions will be medically useful. The others, usually weaker effects, are called side effects. They are not necessarily harmful, but may be annoying.

STIMULANT. Any of several drugs which act on the central nervous system, producing excitation, alertness, and wakefulness. Medical uses include the treatment of mild depressive states, overweight, and narcolepsy—a disease characterized by an almost overwhelming desire to sleep.

SYNERGISM. Action of two agencies which results in a total effect greater than the sum of the two effects taken independently.

TOLERANCE. With many drugs, a person must keep increasing the dosage to maintain the same effect. This characteristic is called tolerance. Tolerance develops with the barbiturates, with amphetamine and related compounds, and with opiates.

TOXIC EFFECTS (poisoning). Any substance in excessive amounts can act as a poison or toxin. With drugs, the margin between the dosage that produces beneficial effects and dosage that produces toxic or poisonous effects varies greatly. Moreover, this margin will vary with the person taking the drug.

Index